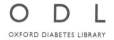

ODL
OXFORD DIABETES LIBRARY

T0200116

# Diabetic Retinopathy: Screening to Treatment

# O D L
OXFORD DIABETES LIBRARY

# Diabetic Retinopathy: Screening to Treatment

Second Edition

Edited by

## Ramesh R. Sivaraj, MS, DNB, FRCS Ed, FRCOphth

Consultant Ophthalmologist and Honorary Senior Lecturer,
Department of Ophthalmology, University Hospitals Birmingham
NHS Foundation Trust, and Honorary Senior Lecturer,
Department of Optometry, Aston University, Birmingham,
West Midlands, UK

## Paul M. Dodson, MD, FRCP, FRCOphth

Honorary Professor Aston University
Department of Life Sciences,
and Warwick Medical School
Clinical Science Research Institute, UK,
and Addis Ababa University, Ethiopia;
Consultant in Diabetes, Ophthalmic Medicine
and Medical Ophthalmology,
University Hospital Birmingham, Birmingham, UK
Chairman of the Board of Trustees,
Oakhaven Hospice, Hampshire UK

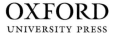

OXFORD
UNIVERSITY PRESS

# OXFORD
UNIVERSITY PRESS

Great Clarendon Street, Oxford, OX2 6DP,
United Kingdom

Oxford University Press is a department of the University of Oxford.
It furthers the University's objective of excellence in research, scholarship,
and education by publishing worldwide. Oxford is a registered trade mark of
Oxford University Press in the UK and in certain other countries

First Edition published in 2008
Second Edition published in 2020

Impression: 1

Published in the United States of America by Oxford University Press
198 Madison Avenue, New York, NY 10016, United States of America

British Library Cataloguing in Publication Data

Data available

Library of Congress Control Number: 2019947975

ISBN 978–0–19–883445–8

Printed and bound by
CPI Group (UK) Ltd, Croydon, CR0 4YY

# Preface

As the epidemic of diabetes unfolds, the need for additional treatments and strategies to limit diabetic complications becomes ever more pressing. While research continues into new therapies, the feared complications of diabetes are still too common across the world, with blindness the number one for many patients.

Newer therapies, such as anti-vascular endothelial growth factor (anti-VEGF) and steroid implants in addition to laser treatment, has reduced visual loss, but needs to be considered early. Screening has helped pick up diabetic retinopathy (DR) and maculopathy at an early asymptomatic stage, bestowing maximum treatment benefit.

The UK has successfully run a DR screening programme using digital technology, encompassing the four nations of England, Wales, Scotland, and Northern Ireland since 2006, comparable with cervical and breast cancer screening. The considerable investment and continued funding in both capital equipment and recruitment of new staff, including photographers, screeners, graders, optometrists, nurses, administrators, commissioners, and clinicians in diabetes and ophthalmology has helped this develop well. It has reduced the incidence of sight impairment related to diabetes by about a half.

This pocketbook aims to be a concise companion for those professionals involved in the DR screening programme, which is now a NVQ Level 3 Health Screener Qualification. The pocket size of this book does not allow for an exhaustive description of every aspect of DR or the differences between the four nations' screening programmes. It is a summary of the basis of screening and practical information, with no intention of diminishing the important variations in schemes, e.g. in grading levels, numbers of photographs taken per eye, and the use of mydriasis.

The book covers the basics of diabetes mellitus and ocular anatomy for those new to the subject, leading onto why screening is required, the epidemiology, and nature of DR and associated ocular diseases.

The second edition includes descriptions of recent changes in national screening, grading, and administration, with final sections on advances in imaging and treatment of DR, from both medical and ophthalmological perspectives, which have evolved significantly since the first edition was published. It also includes a brief discussion on a new era of artificial intelligence and deep learning algorithms which are set to revolutionize the way screening might be done in the future. A section is included on the important area of information technology that underpins computers, digital imaging, connectivity, and servers. An appendix discusses the different grading systems used in other parts of the world, and describes some of the differences to the UK screening programme.

The authors hope this concise companion will not only inform staff in the UK system, but also those in diabetic screening programmes across the world, particularly those in gestation in establishing national programmes.

We are very grateful to our Consultant colleagues (Professor Jonathan Gibson, Ms Sarita Jacob, Ms Sobha Joseph, Dr Alexander Wright, and Dr Margaret Clarke) and all the contributors to the book who are a part of the Birmingham and Black Country Diabetic Retinopathy Screening Programme, who have done sterling work with the first and second editions.

The authors would also like to thank all those at Oxford University Press for making this book possible, to Karen Whitehouse and Helen Wharton for editorial assistance, and our families (Renu, Rohit, and Sanjana Ramesh) and (Lynne, James, Alex, and Ellie Dodson) for their continual support.

Ramesh R. Sivaraj and Paul M. Dodson

# Contents

# Abbreviations

| | |
|---|---|
| 1DD | one disc diameter |
| AAA | abdominal aortic aneurysm |
| ACE | angiotensin-converting enzyme |
| ACCORD | Action to Control Cardiovascular Risk in Diabetes |
| AGE | advanced glycation end products |
| AI | artificial intelligence |
| AMD | age-related macular degeneration |
| ARB | angiotensin receptor blocker |
| BARS | British Association of Retinal Screening |
| BCSP | bowel cancer screening programme |
| BMI | body mass index |
| BP | blood pressure |
| BRVO | branch retinal vein occlusion |
| BSP | breast screening programme |
| CARDS | Collaborative Atorvastatin Diabetes Study |
| CF | count fingers |
| CHRPE | congenital hypertrophy of the retinal pigment epithelium |
| CIDMO | central involving diabetic macular oedema |
| CNS | central nervous system |
| CRVO | central retinal vein occlusion |
| CSII | continuous subcutaneous infusion of short-acting insulin |
| cSLO | confocal scanning laser ophthalmoscopy |
| CSMO | clinically significant macular oedema |
| CSP | cervical screening programme |
| CWS | cotton wool spots |
| DCCT | Diabetes Control and Complications Trial |
| DD | disc diameter |
| DES | diabetic eye screening |
| DESP | diabetic eye screening programme |
| DL | deep learning |
| DMO | diabetic macular oedema |
| DR | diabetic retinopathy |
| DRS | Diabetic Retinopathy Study |
| DS | digital surveillance |
| ECG | electrocardiogram |

| | |
|---|---|
| EDI | enhanced depth imaging |
| EDIC | Epidemiology of Diabetes Interventions and Complications |
| EQA | external quality assurance |
| ERM | epi-retinal membrane |
| ESR | erythrocyte sedimentation ratio |
| ETDRS | Early Treatment Diabetic Retinopathy Study |
| EUCLID | EURODIAB Controlled Trial of Lisinopril in Insulin-Dependent Diabetes |
| FASP | foetal anomaly screening programme |
| FBC | full blood count |
| FFA | fundus fluorescein angiography |
| FGF | fibroblast growth factor |
| FIELD | Fenofibrate Intervention and Event Lowering in Diabetes |
| GH | growth hormone |
| GFR | glomerular filtration rate |
| GOC | General Optical Council |
| GTT | glucose tolerance test |
| HbA1C | glycated haemoglobin |
| HDL | high density lipoprotein |
| HES | hospital eye service |
| HM | hand movements |
| IDPS | infectious diseases in pregnancy screening programme |
| IGF-1 | insulin-like growth factor-1 |
| IQA | internal quality assessment |
| IRMA | intra-retinal microvascular abnormalities |
| IT | information technology |
| iTAT | international test and training |
| KPI | key performance indicator |
| LADA | latent autoimmune diabetes of adults |
| LASER | light amplification by stimulated emission of radiation |
| LDL | low density lipoprotein |
| M1 | maculopathy |
| MODY | maturity diabetes of the young |
| NBS | newborn blood spot |
| NHSP | newborn hearing screening programme |
| NHSDESP | NHS Diabetic Eye Screening Programme |
| NIPE | newborn and infant physical examination |
| NPDR | non-proliferative diabetic retinopathy |
| NPL | no perception of light |
| NSC | National Screening Committee |

| | |
|---|---|
| NVD | new vessels at the optic disc |
| NVE | new vessels elsewhere |
| OCT | optical coherence tomography |
| OCTA | optical coherence tomography angiography |
| OD | optics disc |
| OSA | obstructive sleep apnoea |
| PASCAL | patterned-scanning laser |
| PDR | proliferative diabetic retinopathy |
| PGD | patient group directive |
| PHE | Public Health England |
| PKC | protein kinase C |
| PL | perception of light |
| POAG | primary open angle glaucoma |
| PRP | pan-retinal photocoagulation |
| QA | quality assurance |
| RAO | retinal artery occlusion |
| RAS | renin–angiotensin system |
| RDS | routine annual digital screening |
| ROG | referral outcome grader |
| RPE | retinal pigment epithelium |
| RPL | recognition of prior learning |
| RVO | retinal vein occlusion |
| sc | subcutaneous |
| SCL | single collated list |
| SCT | sickle cell and thalassaemia |
| SD | spectral domain |
| SLB | slit lamp biomicroscopy |
| SQAS | screening quality assurance service |
| STDR | sight-threatening diabetic retinopathy |
| SVL | severe visual loss |
| TD | time domain |
| TFT | thyroid function test |
| U&E | urea and electrolytes |
| UKPDS | United Kingdom Prospective Diabetes Study |
| UWF | ultra-wide field |
| VA | visual acuity |
| VAP | vascular adhesion protein |
| VEGF | vascular endothelial growth factor |
| VPN | virtual private network |

# Contributors

**Prashant Amrelia**

Bachelor of Science, Slit Lamp Examiner and Grader, Diabetic Eye Screening, University Hospitals Birmingham, Birmingham, West Midlands, UK

**Paul M. Dodson**

Honorary Professor Aston University Department of Life Sciences, and Warwick Medical School Clinical Science Research Institute UK, and Addis Ababa University, Ethiopia; Consultant in Diabetes, Ophthalmic Medicine and Medical Ophthalmology, University Hospital Birmingham, Birmingham, UK Chairman of the Board of Trustees, Oakhaven Hospice, Hampshire UK

**Navjot K. Gahir**

Diabetic Retinopathy Screener/Grader, Diabetes and Endocrinology Centre, University Hospitals Birmingham, Birmingham, West Midlands, UK

**Paul Galsworthy**

Joint Programme and Grading Centre Manager, Diabetic Eye Screening, University Hospitals Birmingham, Birmingham, West Midlands, UK

**Jonathan M. Gibson**

Emeritus Professor of Ophthalmology, School of Life and Health Science, Aston University, Birmingham, West Midlands, UK

**Sarita Jacob**

Consultant Ophthalmologist and Hon Senior Clinical Lecturer, Ophthalmology, University Hospitals of Birmingham and University of Birmingham, Birmingham, West Midlands, UK

**Sobha Joseph**

Consultant, Ophthalmology, University Hospitals of Birmingham NHS Trust and Visiting Senior Lecturer, School of Life and Health Sciences, Aston University, Birmingham, West Midlands, UK

**Andrew Mills**

IT Manager, Diabetic Eye Screening, University Hospital Birmingham NHS Foundation Trust, Birmingham, West Midlands, UK

**David K. Roy**

Clinical Governance Manager, Slit Lamp Examiner, Diabetic Eye Screening, University Hospitals Birmingham, Birmingham, West Midlands, UK

**Mirriam Shah**

Slit Lamp Examiner and Grader, Diabetic Eye Screening, University Hospitals Birmingham, West Midlands, UK

**Emma Shepherd**

Diabetic Screener/Grader, Diabetic Eye Screening, University Hospitals Birmingham, Birmingham, West Midlands, UK

**Ramesh R. Sivaraj**

Consultant Ophthalmologist and Honorary Senior Lecturer, Department of Ophthalmology, University Hospitals Birmingham NHS Foundation Trust, and Department of Optometry, Aston University, Birmingham, West Midlands, UK

**Rebecca Smith**

Joint Programme and Failsafe Manager,
Diabetic Eye Screening, University
Hospitals Birmingham, Birmingham,
West Midlands, UK

**Rachel Stockwin**

Diabetic Screener/Grader, Diabetic
Eye Screening, University Hospitals
Birmingham, Birmingham,
West Midlands, UK

**Helen Wharton**

Senior Diabetic Eye Screener/Grader,
Diabetic Eye Screening, University
Hospitals Birmingham, Birmingham,
West Midlands, UK

**Karen Whitehouse**

Senior Diabetic Retinopathy Grader,
Education Manager, Diabetic Eye
Screening, University Hospitals
Birmingham, Birmingham,
West Midlands, UK

**Alexander D. Wright**

Consultant Diabetologist, Diabetes
Department, University Hospitals
Birmingham, Birmingham,
West Midlands, UK

# CHAPTER 1

# What is diabetes?

Alexander D. Wright

**KEY POINTS**

- The definition of diabetes is based on an increased concentration of glucose in the blood.
- The basic defect is a relative or absolute lack of the hormone insulin, which promotes the uptake of glucose into tissues.
- Insulin is made in islets within the pancreas gland.
- A familial tendency is often found.
- Type 1 diabetes is due to autoimmune destruction of the islets and insulin therapy is essential.
- Type 2 diabetes is due to a relative lack of insulin, often with tissue insulin resistance; diet and lifestyle changes are often effective initially but, as the condition progresses, oral therapy and insulin are usually required eventually.
- All forms of diabetes are associated with long-term vascular complications affecting both small and large arteries.

## 1.1 Introduction

Diabetes mellitus is an increasingly common metabolic disorder, affecting 6% of the UK population and using 10% of health resources, sometimes referred to as sugar diabetes, or more graphically, as the pissing evil. Diabetes is the common term used to describe the condition. The adjective 'diabetic' can be used to describe, for example, diabetic retinopathy, but should not to be used to describe a patient or an object, such as a clinic, but rather they should be described as 'a patient with diabetes' or 'diabetes clinic'. The number affected may rise to 5 million by 2030 unless prevention programmes become effective. Most diabetes tends to run in families and an increase in genetically predisposed individuals in the UK may explain part of the rise in prevalence, but changes in factors such as an increase in obesity and reduction in physical exercise are probably more important.

## 1.2 Basic defect

The basic defect in diabetes is a relative or absolute lack of insulin—a peptide hormone produced by the beta cells in the islets of Langerhans scattered throughout the pancreas gland. Insulin is essential for storing glucose by promoting the transfer of glucose from the blood into muscle and liver (as glycogen) and into fatty tissues (as fat). The concentration of glucose in the blood is very tightly controlled, between approximately 5 and 10 mmol/L. Without insulin glucose levels rise and glucose is excreted into the urine. The classic symptoms of diabetes are therefore weight loss, tiredness, thirst, excessive urination (especially noted at night, including bed-wetting in children), and genital irritation (thrush). Sometimes vision becomes blurred. Brain and nervous tissues are not generally affected by high blood glucose concentrations, but malfunction when glucose level falls below 4.0 mmol as a result of treatment, with a group of symptoms collectively referred to as a 'hypo'.

## 1.3 Diagnosis

Diabetes may be suspected by the finding of glucose in the urine, but is diagnosed as a fasting plasma concentration of ≥7.0 mmol/L (126 mg/dL), or a 2-hour post-glucose load plasma glucose of ≥11.1 mmol/L (200 mg/dL), or glycated haemoglobin, HbA1C of ≥48 mmol/mol (6.5%; see Table 1.1). Blood should be freshly drawn, delivered without delay, and measured in a laboratory. A second measurement should be obtained to confirm the diagnosis in patients without symptoms, or if there is a marked discrepancy between the plasma glucose concentrations and HbA1C (see Box 1.1). If a marked discrepancy persists, an abnormality in haemoglobin or its turnover should be considered.

## 1.4 Types of diabetes

The different types of diabetes describe a wide range of the condition and its causes. This should not overly concern the retinal screener as the terms are not always used correctly by health professionals or by patients. More importantly, retinopathy may occur in all types of diabetes, therefore justifying its inclusion in screening all programmes, the only exception being gestational diabetes.

Type 1 diabetes (previously known as insulin-dependent or juvenile-onset diabetes) is due to autoimmune destruction of the beta cells in the pancreas. In many patients, auto-antibodies against islet peptides can be detected. A number of gene associations has been found and there is a considerable worldwide variation in incidence ranging from <1.0/100,000 in Mexico, Korea, China, Peru, and Tanzania,

| Table 1.1 Definition of degrees of glucose intolerance | | |
|---|---|---|
| Venous plasma glucose (mmol/L) | Overnight fast | 2-hour post-glucose load |
| Diabetes mellitus | ≥7.0 | and/or ≥11.1 |
| Impaired glucose tolerance | <7.0 | and ≥7.8 to <11.1 |
| Impaired fasting glycaemia | ≥6.0 to <7.0 | if measured <7.8 |

---

**Box 1.1** Diagnostic pathway for diabetes

- *Think* of the diagnosis if excessive thirst and passing of urine, weight loss, tiredness, incontinence, vulval or penile rash, foot ulcer, or blurred vision.
- *Suspect* diagnosis if urine positive for glucose.
- *Confirm* diagnosis by measuring glucose level in blood; test urine for ketones if positive for glucose; glucose tolerance test (GTT) involves an overnight fast and drinking 75 g glucose.
- *Diagnosis* of diabetes symptoms + blood glucose >7.0 fasting or 11.1 mmol/L post-meal, or no symptoms and abnormal blood glucose on two separate occasions.
- *Consider* the diagnosis of Type 1 diabetes if abnormal blood glucose *and* moderate or heavy ketonuria. Sometimes antibodies are measured to confirm an autoimmune process.
- *Consider* the diagnosis of Type 2 diabetes if abnormal blood glucose, *but* no or light ketonuria.
- *Consider* a genetic form if Type 2 diabetes occurs in a young person.

---

to 36/10,000 in Finland. It occurs more commonly in children, often presenting acutely, but can occur at any age with a slower rate of onset in adults (sometime known as latent autoimmune diabetes of adults [LADA]). Insulin treatment is essential for Type 1 diabetes. Insulin deficiency is also found, but without antibodies in young people, mainly of African or Asian descent, who suffer episodic uncontrolled diabetes (ketoacidosis) and a variable need for insulin treatment.

Type 2 diabetes (previously known as non-insulin-dependent diabetes or adult-onset diabetes) is caused by a relative lack of insulin, often associated with tissue insulin resistance. Unlike Type 1 diabetes, patients do not require insulin to survive, at least in the first few years of the condition. Nevertheless, the condition tends to be progressive, and insulin treatment is often required, thus becoming insulin-treated Type 2 diabetes (but *not* Type 1 diabetes). Type 2 diabetes can be found at any age, but is more common in middle-aged or elderly people. Predisposing risk factors are certain racial/ethnic groups, being overweight (body mass index [BMI] ≥23–25 depending on racial group), and lack of physical activity; some associated conditions include hypertension, polycystic ovaries, certain medications (glucocorticoid steroids, diuretics, anti-psychotics, drugs used in organ transplantation, anti-viral drugs), and pancreatic diseases (for example, cystic fibrosis, pancreatitis, haemochromatosis, pancreatectomy). Diabetes may develop in pregnancy (gestational diabetes), but usually reverts to normal after delivery; however, such patients remain at significant risk of developing Type 2 diabetes in the future. Retinopathy screening is not normally advocated in patients with gestational diabetes, or indeed in patients with 'pre-diabetes' (those at risk of developing diabetes).

Other types of diabetes include monogenic diabetes (maturity diabetes of the young [MODY]), neonatal diabetes, and diabetes as a part of other genetic syndromes. A prospective study of patients with newly diagnosed diabetes in Scandinavia largely confirmed these traditional subdivisions. In addition to auto-antibodies, insulin secretion and resistance were measured, and patients were sub-divided into five clusters. From a retinal screening point of view, no difference was found in the five clusters in the time to diabetic retinopathy.

## 1.5 Complications

Complications may be acute due to very high blood glucose concentrations (diabetic coma or ketoacidosis), or abnormally low blood glucose concentrations (hypoglycaemia), or more long-term over several years due to damage to capillary vessels (microvascular) or arteries (macrovascular), or other direct tissue damage.

## 1.6 Principles of treatment

Education on diabetes and its consequences soon after diagnosis and subsequently is a vital part of management. Therapy aims to restore effective insulin action, maintain blood glucose concentration within the normal range of ~5–10 mmol/L, and avoid long-term complications (see Box 1.2). Principles of dietary therapy include avoidance of simple carbohydrates (glucose and sucrose), appropriate distribution of complex carbohydrates, and maintenance of normal body weight (see Box 1.3). Drug therapy may be relatively simple initially, but tends to become more complex in diabetes of long duration.

Self-monitoring is performed on capillary blood with blood glucose strips or on tissue glucose by implanted glucose sensitive devices. Laboratory testing involves measurement of the amount of glucose attached to the haemoglobin

---

**Box 1.2** Long-term complications of diabetes

- *Macrovascular (large vessel)*:
  - o *Coronary*—angina, heart attacks, heart failure.
  - o *Carotid and cerebral*—strokes, disturbance of vision.
  - o *Peripheral vessels*—pain on walking, foot ulceration, gangrene.
- *Microvascular (small vessel)*:
  - o *Eye*—retinopathy (cataracts, glaucoma also more common).
  - o *Kidney (nephropathy)*—leaking of albumin in the urine, nephrotic syndrome, renal failure.
  - o *Nervous system (neuropathy)*—peripheral nerve damage, muscle wasting, cranial nerve palsies, autonomic nerve damage.
- *Skin*: fungal infections, carbuncles and pyoderma gangrenosum, necrobiosis lipoidica diabeticorum.
- *Joints*: stiffness of the fingers, Charcot (neuropathic) joints, frozen shoulder.

> **Box 1.3** Basic management of diabetes
>
> - Diet, lifestyle (exercise, no smoking), weight loss if obese.
> - *Improve insulin sensitivity*: oral metformin or thiazolidinedione.
> - *Stimulate insulin secretion*: oral sulphonylureas, metiglinides, incretins (oral or injectable).
> - *Increase urine excretion of glucose*: oral gliflocins.
> - *Replace insulin*:
>   - subcutaneous (sc) injections (1–5 times a day, depending on the type of insulin); short-acting insulin to cover meals and long-acting insulin to cover basal needs;
>   - continuous sc infusion of short-acting insulin (CSII) 'insulin pump';
> - Monitoring blood glucose, blood pressure (BP), and lipids.
> - Observe eyes, feet, and kidney function.

(glycated haemoglobin or HbA1C). In the absence of any disturbance of red cells or haemoglobin, this is a useful measure of glycaemic control over the previous 6 weeks. Normal HbA1C is <42 mmol/mol with borderline results 42–48 mmol/mol. Target levels are ≤56 mmol/mol. If there are changes in red cells or haemoglobin, falsely high or low readings of HbA1C may be obtained, and an alternative measure of serum fructosamine may be helpful. The laboratory is also required for measurement of protein in the urine (albumin/creatinine ratio).

## 1.7 Summary

Diabetes mellitus is characterized by increases in concentrations of glucose, and diagnosed by a fasting plasma glucose concentration of ≥7.0 mmol/L (126 mg/dL), or a 2-hour post-glucose load of ≥11.1 mmol/L (200 mg/dL), or glycated haemoglobin, HbA1C ≥48 mmol/mol (6.5%). Type 1 diabetes is due to an autoimmune destruction of the insulin producing cells in the islets in the pancreas and requires treatment with insulin. Type 2 diabetes is caused by a combination of insulin resistance and the gradual failure of insulin production, and can often be managed by dietary and lifestyle methods initially, but later may require oral medications and insulin. Long-term complications may occur in any patient with diabetes, and can include disease of large and small vessels.

FURTHER READING

Ahlqvist E, Storm P, Käräjämäki A, Martinell M, Dorkan M, Carlson A, et al. (2018). Novel subgroups of adult-onset diabetes and their association with outcomes: a data-driven cluster analysis of six variables. *Lancet Diabetes Endocrinol* **6**: 361–9.

American Diabetes Association Position Statement. (2018). Classification and diagnosis of diabetes. *Diabetes Care* **41**(Suppl. 1): S13–27.

Davies MJ, D'Alessio DA, Fradkin J, Walter N, Kernan WN, Chantal Mathieu C, et al. (2018). Management of hyperglycaemia in type 2 diabetes, 2018. A consensus report by the American Diabetes Association (ADA) and the European Association for the Study of Diabetes (EASD). *Diabetologia* **61**: 2461–89.

NICE. Diabetes (type 1 and type 2) in children and young people: diagnosis and management, NICE guideline NG18. https://www.nice.org.uk/guidance/ng18 (accessed 7 August 2019).

NICE. Equality and Human Rights Consultation. Type 2 diabetes in adults: Management, Nice guideline NG28. https://www.health-ni.gov.uk/consultations/equality-and-human-rights-consultation-nice-ng-28-type-2-diabetes-adults-management (accessed 7 August 2019).

NICE. Type 1 diabetes in adults: diagnosis and management, NICE guideline NG17. https://www.nice.org.uk/guidance/ng17 (accessed 7 August 2019).

# CHAPTER 2

# Diabetic retinopathy: reasons for screening

Paul Galsworthy

---

---

## 2.1 Introduction

At the time of writing, there are roughly 3.7 million people diagnosed with diabetes in the UK and over 12 million are at an increased risk of Type 2 diabetes. Diabetes and its associated complications costs the NHS £10 billion a year, roughly 10% of the total NHS budget; this equates to £17,000 a minute spent on diabetes care. Much of this money is spent on patients requiring hospital admittance to treat diabetes-related complications. There needs to be a move towards prevention, rather than cure.

Diabetic retinopathy (DR) is a microvascular (small vessel) disease affecting the retinal vasculature, leading to progressive retinal damage, which may lead to sight loss or even blindness. Despite advances in DES, diabetes management, and widely available laser and intra-vitreal injections for treating eye disease DR, associated visual loss is still all too common for the following reasons:

- Late presentation for eye screening and/or treatment (patients are often asymptomatic until eye disease is at an advanced stage).
- Poor engagement in diabetes care.
- Not all cases of maculopathy and proliferative retinopathy respond to laser or intra-vitreal treatment.

## 2.2 Causes of visual loss in people with diabetes

Diabetic eye disease is a group of eye conditions that can cause vision loss and blindness among people with diabetes. These conditions include DR/macular oedema, cataracts, and glaucoma.

It is estimated that within 20 years of diagnosis, nearly all patients with Type 1 diabetes and 60% of Type 2 patients will have DR.

Every year, over 1500 people are certified as visually impaired or severely visually impaired in England and Wales as a result of DR.

It is well established that people are at increased risk of developing DR with high glucose, blood pressure (BP), and cholesterol levels. However, more recent studies also concluded that there are strong links associated with deprivation and within ethnic minority groups.

People with diabetes are twice as likely to develop glaucoma and are more likely to develop cataracts at an earlier age, as diabetes also affects the lens of the eye. It is therefore important that patients have both refractive eye tests with optometrists, but also attend regular DES. The importance of the two separate tests should be explained to patients as DES alone is not sufficient eye health care.

Between 5 and 10% of people will develop proliferative DR, although it is more common in people with Type 1 diabetes than Type 2. Maculopathy is the major cause of vision loss, particularly in people with Type 2 diabetes.

However, the causes of blindness in people with diabetes can also be due to other conditions, particularly as people with Type 2 diabetes are generally older and may have other ocular diseases.

Non-diabetic retinopathy causes of visual loss in diabetic subjects include:

- Inherited eye disease:
  - glaucoma;
  - age-related macular degeneration (AMD);
  - retinitis pigmentosa;
  - optic atrophy.
- Trauma and injury.
- Amblyopia.
- Retinal vein or artery occlusions, ischaemic optic neuropathy.
- Cataracts.
- Hypertension (and macro-aneurysms).
- Retinal detachment.
- Retinal dystrophies and myopic degeneration.

While detecting DR is the primary purpose of the diabetic eye screening programme (DESP), non-diabetic eye conditions detected will require individual providers to produce clear protocols and pathways to ensure they are managed appropriately.

## 2.3 Does diabetic eye screening reduce visual loss

DR is no longer the leading cause of blindness in the working-age population; this is now inherited eye diseases. Although the number of people with diabetes has risen, the rate of blindness from DR has not. Recent data have confirmed that between 2007 and 2015 there was a 43% reduction of newly recorded certifications of visual impairment due to DR in Wales; this is among the first data since the introduction of the national DESP in 2006 to demonstrate substantial benefit. This may, in part, be due to the ability of DESP to detect disease at an early stage successfully when the disease responds better to treatment, and in part to increased treatment options now available to clinicians which are more successful.

Together with advances in general diabetes care, a far greater choice of medication options for patients in the form of oral tablets, insulin, or non-insulin injection options are available to treat glucose levels, BP, and cholesterol.

The cost of blindness or partial sightedness is considerable in terms of social and welfare costs, but also in loss of income during working life (£20,000 per patient registered blind per year). Indeed, visual loss is one of the most feared complications of diabetes by patients.

Both in Europe and the USA, national bodies have assessed the cost effectiveness of a DR screening programme, and have concluded that screening saves vision for a relatively low cost and even this cost is often less than the disability payments provided to people who would go blind in the absence of a screening programme (American Diabetes Association statement 1998).

## 2.4 Definition of screening

The National Screening Committee (NSC) defines screening as a 'public service in which members of a defined population who do not necessarily perceive they are at risk of or are already affected by a disease or its complications, are asked a question or offered a test to identify those individuals who are more likely to be helped than harmed by further tests or treatment to reduce the risk of a disease or its complications'.

The criteria for a successful screening programme are described by Wilson and Jungner (1968):

- The condition sought should be an important health problem.
- There should be an accepted treatment for patients with recognized disease.
- Facilities for diagnosis and treatment should be available.
- There should be a recognizable latent or early symptomatic stage.
- Screening for disease:
  ○ There should be a suitable test or examination.
  ○ The test should be acceptable to the population.

○ The natural history of the condition, including development from latent to declared disease, should be adequately understood.

○ There should be an agreed policy on whom to treat as patients.

○ The cost of case-finding (including diagnosis and treatment of patients diagnosed) should be economically balanced in relation to possible expenditure on medical care as a whole.

○ Case-finding should be a continuing process and not a 'once and for all' project.

Source: adapted from Wilson & Jungner. https://www.who.int/
bulletin/volumes/86/4/07-050112/en/.

Screening for DR using digital imaging fulfils these requirements for a screening programme. DR has important adverse effects, and while laser and intra-vitreal treatment is effective, it can be easily detected by digital imaging, which is an acceptable test and is cost effective.

## 2.5 Population screening

A number of national screening programmes spanning the four nations of the UK have been established and these include:

- NHS abdominal aortic aneurysm (AAA) programme.
- NHS bowel cancer screening programme (BCSP).
- NHS breast screening programme (BSP).
- NHS cervical screening programme (CSP).
- NHS diabetic eye screening programme (NHSDESP).
- NHS foetal anomaly screening programme (FASP).
- NHS infectious diseases in pregnancy screening programme (IDPS).
- NHS newborn and infant physical examination (NIPE) screening programme.
- NHS newborn blood spot (NBS) screening programme.
- NHS newborn hearing screening programme (NHSP).
- NHS sickle cell and thalassaemia (SCT) screening programme.

With regard to DES, the four nations operate slightly differently in their model, delivery, and IT systems, although all follow set policies and guidelines to ensure a safe and efficient programme.

A screening programme can only truly be effective if its defined population is undertaking the test and receiving the necessary treatment if required.

At the time of writing, the current uptake for the DESP is approximately 82%, although this meets the current standard set of a minimum of 75% across England. Of concern, this equates to approximately 500,000 patients not undertaking annual DES, who will be at risk of DR if left undetected and thereby untreated.

FURTHER READING

Garvican L, Clowes J, Gillow T. (2000). Preservation of sight in diabetes; developing a national risk reduction programme *Diabet Med* **17**: 627–34.

Thomas RL, Luzio SD, North RV, Banerjee S, Zekite A, Bunce C, et al. (2017). Retrospective analysis of newly recorded certifications of visual impairment due to diabetic retinopathy in Wales during 2007–2015. *Br Med J Open* **18**(7): e015024.

Wilson JMG, Jungner G. (1968) Principles and practice of screening for disease. WHO, Geneva. https://apps.who.int/iris/handle/10665/37650 (accessed 29 August 2019).

# Anatomy of the eye and the healthy fundus

Navjot K. Gahir and Mirriam Shah

**KEY POINTS**

- The human eye is an intricate and widely used major sense organ of the body. It can be divided into two main segments—the anterior segment and the posterior segment.
- This chapter describes and includes pictorial emphasis of the anatomy of the eye and, more specifically, the structure and function of the retina.

## 3.1 The anterior segment

The anterior segment makes up the front third of the eye. It includes the cornea, iris, ciliary body, lens, and two fluid spaces filled with aqueous humour—the anterior chamber and the posterior chamber (see Figure 3.1).

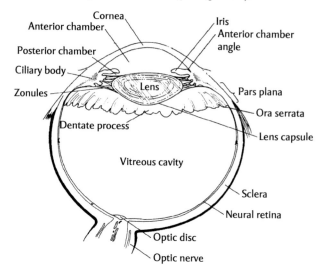

Figure 3.1 Cross-section of the human eye.
Reproduced courtesy of Professor Paul M. Dodson and The Heart of England Retinal Screening Centre.

The anterior chamber is the space between the innermost surface of the cornea, and the anterior surfaces of the iris and lens.

### 3.1.1 The cornea

The cornea is a transparent 'window'-like protective layer at the front of the eye. The size of the cornea is approximately 11.5 mm in diameter. The cornea plays an important role in focusing vision. Both the cornea and the lens refract light, enabling the eye to focus. The cornea contributes more to the total refraction but, unlike the lens, the curvature of the cornea is not fixed and cannot be adjusted to refine the focus. The cornea, together with the sclera, makes up the outermost layer of the eyeball, forming a durable, protective barrier that helps shield against any trauma or infection, and serves as a defence against the invasion of microorganisms and foreign material into the eye.

### 3.1.2 The sclera

The sclera is commonly known as the 'white' of the eye. It makes up the spherical outer wall of the eyeball and is continuous right up to the edge of the cornea. The thickness of the sclera can vary from approximately 0.3 to 1 mm. Its main functions include protecting against internal and external forces, acting as a type of connective tissue, and providing attachment for the muscles exterior to the globe of the eye. The sclera is strengthened by collagen fibrils, allowing it to maintain the global shape of the eye.

### 3.1.3 The iris

This is the most coloured and visible part of the eye surrounding the pupil. The iris can be strongly pigmented and consists of tissue known as stroma. The colours can vary between blue, brown, green, grey, and hazel. At the centre of the iris is the pupil, an aperture that can become smaller (contract), using a sphincter muscle running radially through the iris, connected to the stroma, or become larger (dilate), due to a dilator muscle, also connected to the stroma.

The iris has two main functions—controlling light entry to the retina and reducing light scatter. Therefore, the iris regulates the amount of light that enters the eye by being able to adjust the size of the pupil opening.

### 3.1.4 The lens

The lens is found in the anterior segment of the eye; it is a flexible, transparent biconvex structure and helps to refract light. Its main purpose is to reflect light onto the back of the eye (retina), along with the help of the cornea, and its transparency is achieved due to the fact that it is acellular and most of the layers of the lens have the same index refraction.

By altering the lens curvature, the eye is able to focus on objects at different distances from it. The curvature of the lens is changed and controlled by the circularly arranged ciliary muscle, situated in the uveal part of the ciliary body. Zonular fibres arise from the ciliary body and are inserted into the zonule in the lens, suspending it in position during accommodation. This enables changes in the ciliary muscle to affect lens curvature.

For short-range focus, the ciliary muscle contracts, releasing tension on the lens caused by zonular fibres, making the lens more convex. For long-range focus, the ciliary muscle relaxes, causing the zonular fibres to become flexed and taut, flattening the lens.

### 3.1.5 The aqueous humour

This is a thick transparent fluid that fills the anterior segment of the eye, which is the space between the cornea and the lens. The aqueous humour has a vital role in the health of the eye. It contributes to the normal maintenance of intra-ocular pressure and helps maintain the convex shape of the cornea. This fluid also contributes to the nutrition of the endothelial layer of the cornea.

The aqueous humour supplies the metabolism of the lens (which is avascular) and carries away the associated waste products. It is secreted by the ciliary processes into the posterior chamber, and flows around the margin of the pupil and into the anterior chamber.

Around 80% of the aqueous humour drains out from the eye via the trabecular network in the anterior chamber angle, into the canal of Sclemm. Elsewhere, the aqueous humour is also able to flow via the uveoscleral outflow path, into the potential space between the sclera and ciliary body.

## 3.2 The posterior segment

The posterior segment includes the vitreous humour, retina, choroid, and optic nerve (see Figure 3.1).

### 3.2.1 The vitreous humour

This is a colourless gel mass that fills the eye between the lens and retina, contributing to 80% of the globe of the eye with an average volume of 4 mL. Predominantly, it consists of water (99%), and a mixture of collagen, proteins, salts, and sugars. Its main role is to provide a cushioned support and help maintain the spherical shape of the eye.

### 3.2.2 The retina

Traditionally, the retina is said to be made up of 10 layers (Figure 3.2 and Table 3.1). It is a photo-sensitive tissue and heavily involved in sight. It contains many nerve cells that are responsible for sending electrical impulses to the brain via the optic nerve, which forms an image of what we see around us. It covers the inner surface of the eyeball. Overall, it is made up of two main layers, the neurosensory layer and the retinal pigment epithelium (RPE). The neurosensory layer contains

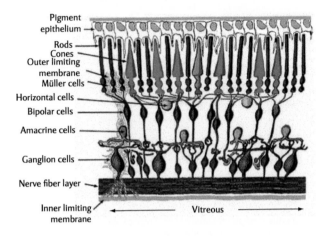

Pigment epithelium
Rods
Cones
Outer limiting membrane
Müller cells
Horizontal cells
Bipolar cells
Amacrine cells
Ganglion cells
Nerve fiber layer
Inner limiting membrane
Vitreous

Figure 3.2 Cross-section layer of the human retina.

Reproduced with permission from Novella S. Suboptimal optics: vision problems as scars of evolutionary history. *Evolution: Education and Outreach*, 1(4): 493–97. © Springer Science+Business Media, LLC 2008. https://doi.org/10.1007/s12052-008-0092-1. Available under the Creative Commons Attribution 4.0 International (CC BY 4.0) http://creativecommons.org/licenses/by/4.0/.

**Table 3.1** The 10 layers of the human retina

| Layer | Description |
|---|---|
| The internal limiting membrane (ILM) | Comprised of Müller cells (glial cells), the ILM serves as a boundary between the retina and vitreous humour. The cells provide support, protection, nutrition, and oxygen to neurons |
| Nerve fibre layer (NFL) | Consists of long, slender projections of neurons, predominantly the axons of retinal ganglion cells and other support cells (amacrine and bipolar cells). Visual information is transmitted along thousands of these nerve fibres from the retina via the rods and cones to the brain, through the optic disc, where they leave the eye |
| Ganglion cells | These cells receive and convey visual information from the photoreceptors to the brain |
| The inner plexiform layer (IPL) | Comprised of axons of bipolar cells and dendrites of neurons from the inner nuclear layer (INL), which are all involved in conducting electrical stimulation |
| The inner nuclear layer (INL) | Contains the nuclei of bipolar neurons, horizontal cells, amacrine cells, and Müller cells |
| The outer plexiform layer (OPL) | Composed of axons, rod, and cone cells, dendrites of bipolar neurons (horizontal cells and amacrine cells), and Müller cells |

| Table 3.1 Continued | |
|---|---|
| Layer | Description |
| The outer nuclear layer (ONL) | Consists of the nuclei of the rod and cone cells |
| The external (outer) limiting membrane (OLM) | Comprises the junction complexes between the Müller cells and rod and cone cells |
| The photoreceptor layer | Responsible for receiving light that reaches the retina. The photoreceptor layer is made up of the outer segments of photoreceptor cells. Cone cells are shorter, darker, and thicker. Rod cells are paler, thinner, and longer |
| Retinal pigment epithelium | (see Section 3.2.5 'The retinal pigment epithelium') |

rods and cones that receive the light, this aids night and peripheral vision, as well as colour and fine detail, respectively. If this area is subject to damage it will most probably affect sight.

### 3.2.3 The neurosensory layer

Overall the neurosensory layer is arranged into three distinct layers:

1. *Internal layer*: contains ganglion cells.
2. *Inner nuclear layer*: contains intermediate neurons.
3. *External layer*: contains the photoreceptor cells.

### 3.2.4 Photoreceptor cells

Photoreceptor cells respond to focused light. There are two types—rod and cone cells.

#### 3.2.4.1 *Rod cells*

Typically, the human retina contains 100 million rod cells; these are more common in the periphery and diminish in number toward the macula. None are found at the fovea and this makes them also responsible for peripheral vision. They have a cylindrical shape and are more sensitive than cone cells. They are responsible for night and low-light vision, and therefore transmit black and white images only.

#### 3.2.4.2 *Cone cells*

Typically, the human retina contains about 7 million cone cells. Cones are present in the highest concentration at the fovea and macula, gradually decreasing in number towards the periphery of the retina. Cone cells are used in fine vision and perception of colour in brighter light. The response time to visual stimuli is faster with cone cells than with rod cells. This makes cone cells able to perceive finer detail and more rapid changes in imagery.

### 3.2.5 The retinal pigment epithelium

The RPE is situated between the photoreceptors and their blood supply, known as the choriocapillaris. It comprises of a single layer of specialist cells known as epithelial cells. These are concerned with the maintenance of the photoreceptors, which involves the removal of waste products. The epithelial cells are hexagonal, making the junctions between them a tight blood barrier.

### 3.2.6 Bruch's membrane

This is the innermost layer of the choroid, which supports the retina. It is made up of five layers:

1. Basement membrane of the RPE.
2. Inner collagenous zone.
3. Central band elastic fibres.
4. Outer collagenous zone.
5. Basement membrane of the choriocapillaris.

The RPE transports metabolic waste products and excess water from the photoreceptors, across the Bruch's membrane to the choroid. This membrane thickens with age, slowing up metabolite transport to the choroid, and this may lead to formation of drusen in age-related macular degeneration (AMD).

### 3.2.7 The choroid

The choroid lies between the retina and the sclera. It contains a supply of blood vessels and pigment. The blood vessels supply nourishment to the outer layers of the retina. The choroid consists of four layers:

1. *Haller's layer*: contains large blood vessels, and is the outermost layer.
2. *Sattler's layer*: contains intermediate-sized blood vessels.
3. *Choriocapillary layer*: contains a layer of capillaries.
4. *Bruch's membrane*: innermost membrane (described previously)

The presence of pigment, dark-coloured melanin, in the choroid helps restrict the amount of internal reflection in the eye by absorbing excess light. The benefits are that clearer images are seen, where otherwise multiple, confused, and/or blurred images would be produced. The red-reflex in retinal photography and red-eye effect in portrait photography is caused by reflection of light from the choroid.

### 3.2.8 The macula

The macula is a highly specialized, functional area of the retina within two disc-diameter of the centre of the fovea. It contains a high proportion of cone cells, which are responsible for visual acuity, colour, and central vision. Therefore, in eye screening, the macula is of particular interest and should always be thoroughly examined for the presence of maculopathy. If the macula and fovea are damaged it is likely to involve major central sight loss in the patient due to the rearrangement and disruption of photoreceptors.

### 3.2.9 The fovea

The fovea is a tiny pit situated at the centre of the macula and is the thinnest part of the retina. It produces the sharpest vision and greatest colour discrimination, due to the high concentration of cone cells. This makes it the part of the eye most involved in central vision, colour, and fine detail. The denser the arrangement of these cone cells, the sharper the vision.

### 3.2.10 The retinal vasculature

The central retinal artery and vein branches out into four main arterial and venous trunks, which run into the nerve fibre layer, supplying each quadrant of the retina with the essential nourishment required to keep it healthy. Therefore, this capillary network of blood vessels is required to keep a constant blood flow within the retina and this is controlled by auto-regulation. This, in turn, is regulated by acute changes in oxygen and major changes in perfusion pressure.

### 3.2.11 The optic nerve

The optic nerve enters the eye through the optic disc. It sends visual information from the eye to the brain and is considered a part of the central nervous system (CNS). It is composed of retinal ganglion cell axons and support cells, and covered with a myelin sheath. The optic nerve contains around 1.2 million nerve fibres, which run from the retina to nine primary visual nuclei in the brain. The eye has a blind spot resulting from the absence of retina at the optic disc

## 3.3 The appearance of a healthy fundus

Retinal appearances differ and colouration varies from intense orange to deeper reddish-brown. It is normal for a fundus to appear lighter and brighter in some places, and duller in others. In terms of layout, the right and left eyes are mirror images of one another, with the optic disc positioned on the nasal side in both eyes.

When looking at a fundus photograph, the side closest to the nose is referred to as nasal and the side furthest away is known as temporal. These terms can either be used to describe regions or 'quadrants' of the fundus.

This example is identifiable as a right eye because the optic disc, which is always on the nasal side, is to the right of the fovea (Figure 3.3). If the photograph were of a left eye, the layout would be close to a mirror image. This means nasal and temporal would be on the opposite sides, and the optic disc would be to the left of the fovea.

The optic disc is the head of the optic nerve and the most obvious feature on the fundus (Figure 3.4). It is yellow in appearance and is about 1.5 mm in diameter. Visible characteristics include a whitish-yellow, funnel-shaped depression called

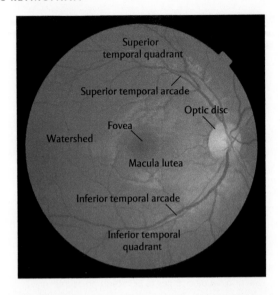

Figure 3.3 **Digital photograph of a healthy fundus (macula-centred view).**
Reproduced courtesy of Professor Paul M. Dodson and The Heart of England Retinal Screening Centre.

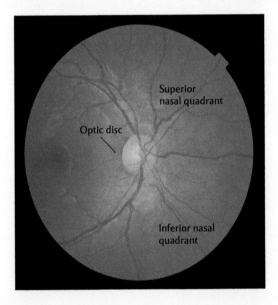

Figure 3.4 **Nasal view of the same fundus, with the optic disc in the centre.**
Reproduced courtesy of Professor Paul M. Dodson and The Heart of England Retinal Screening Centre.

CHAPTER 3

the central cup and a surrounding neural rim. A healthy neural rim is pinkish-orange and has a clearly defined margin.

The optic disc forms a central point for the retinal blood vessels. A superior and inferior arcade, each with arterioles and veins can be seen arching around the fundus, temporal to the optic disc. The pattern and branching of the inferior arcade roughly mirrors that of the superior. The nasal vessels are similarly mirrored, although they simply radiate from the optic disc, as opposed to arching. Finer, single vessels can also be seen at the disc. In a healthy fundus, these follow a logical path without deviating excessively.

Retinal veins appear a deeper red than arteries due to the relative lack of oxygenation in the blood. Temporal to the optic disc is the macula; this is an area appearing darker than the surrounding retina. The main central point of the macula is the fovea.

Understanding the basic anatomy of the human eye is a requirement for all health-care providers, but sound knowledge is of paramount importance to those involved in eye screening.

## 3.4 Normal variations

### 3.4.1 Pigmentation

The colour of the retina is dependent upon ethnicity. Some common examples are shown in Figures 3.5–3.7.

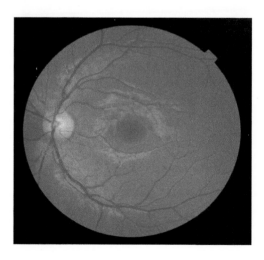

Figure 3.5 **A white, Caucasian fundus (left eye, macula-centred). Typically, these are generally a range of red, orange, and pink tones.**
Reproduced courtesy of Professor Paul M. Dodson and The Heart of England Retinal Screening Centre.

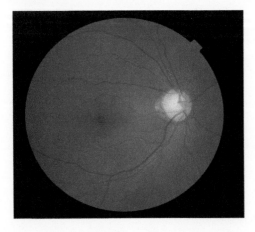

Figure 3.6 A South-Asian fundus (right eye, macula-centred). South-Asian and Afro-Caribbean retinas generally include darker reds and golden browns.
Reproduced courtesy of Professor Paul M. Dodson and The Heart of England Retinal Screening Centre.

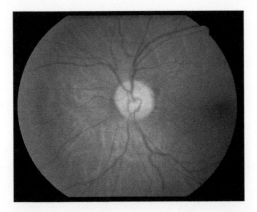

Figure 3.7 Tigroid fundus (left eye, nasal view). The light stripes result from the choroid showing through from beneath the retina, and is common in Afro-Caribbean subjects.
Reproduced courtesy of Professor Paul M. Dodson and The Heart of England Retinal Screening Centre.

## 3.4.2 Glare

Areas of glare or reflection are common in digital fundus photography, particularly around the macula and temporal arcades (Figure 3.8). In appearance, it is pale or translucent, and can range from white-grey to yellow in colour. Glare can usually take the form of delicate, faint, cloud-like patterns or cover whole areas. These are formed as a result of the incoming light from the flash that is necessary for photography. This is more commonly seen in younger individuals as they have a more reflective fundi.

Often, glare can mask or be confused with pathology, meaning extra caution is required. Comparisons between both fields of view can aid a grader to decipher if it is glare resulting from the photography process or actual pathology. If the pale area is not the same in both views or disappears on the other view, then it is generally not remarkable retinopathy.

The variations in the retinal features described above illustrate the array of the normal appearances of a retina. These need to be recognized by all those involved in eye screening to avoid unnecessary referrals and patient anxiety. Other normal variations include tortuosity, myopic crescents, and pseudophakia, which are addressed in other chapters. Experience, exposure, and pattern recognition are paramount to identifying these retinal changes and differentiating them from actual pathology.

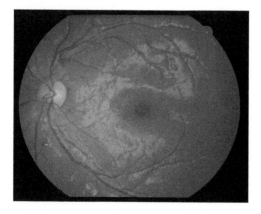

Figure 3.8 **Glare—light patches caused by reflection of camera flash.**
Reproduced courtesy of Professor Paul M. Dodson and The Heart of England Retinal Screening Centre.

FURTHER READING

Dodson PM (ed.). (2008). *Diabetic Retinopathy: screening to treatment*. Oxford University Press, Oxford.

Hughes MO. (2004). Anatomy of the anterior eye for ocularists. *J Ophthalm Prosthet* **2004**: 25–35.

Ng PC, Oliver JJ. (2018). Anatomy of the eye. In: Long B, Koyfman A (eds), *Handbook of Emergency Ophthalmology*, pp. 1–12. Springer, New York.

Snell RS, Lemp MA. (2013). *Clinical anatomy of the eye*. John Wiley & Sons, New York.

Warwick R. (1977). Eugene Wolff's anatomy of the eye and orbit. *Am J Optom Physiolog Optics* **54**(7): 496.

# Diabetes and the eye

Paul M. Dodson

## 4.1 Ocular complications of diabetes

While DR is the most recognized ocular complication, non-DR changes cause up to 50% of cases of blindness in diabetic subjects. Box 4.1 shows the major conditions related to diabetes that occur in clinical practice. It should be noted that the most common cause of blindness in the diabetic population is age-related macular degeneration (AMD).

Type 2 diabetes may present with blurring of vision due to increased myopia (short sight), resulting from overhydration and swelling of the lens, secondary to prolonged hyperglycaemia. These refractive changes reverse as the blood glucose normalizes. It is prudent, however, to delay prescription of glasses for these patients by about 3 months to ensure the metabolic effects are fully resolved.

---

**Box 4.1** Ocular effects of diabetes

Visual change due to:

- Hyperglycaemia leading to refractive changes.
- Cataract.
- DR.
- Background.
- Maculopathy:
  o exudative;
  o ischaemic;
  o mixed exudative and ischaemic;
  o cystoid.
- Pre-proliferative.
- Proliferative.
- Glaucoma:
  o primary open angle;
  o neovascular.
- Cranial nerve palsies (third and sixth nerve) leading to diplopia.
- Retinovascular disease:
  o retinal vein and artery occlusion;
  o ischaemic optic neuropathy.
- Diabetic papillopathy.

---

## 4.2 Cataract

The most common ocular effect of diabetes is of the lens, with resultant cataract formation (see Figure 4.1). This leads to earlier lens opacity formation and more rapid progression. Cataracts affect 60% of older-onset diabetic patients (aged 30–54 years) compared with 12% of non-diabetic controls. There are three main pathogenetic mechanisms. The polyol pathway results in increased glucose conversion by aldose reductase to sorbitol, which sets up an osmotic gradient. This results in movement of water into the cells of the lens, which swells and ruptures with opacity formation. Hyperglycaemia also results in increased glycation of lens proteins and excess free radical formation, leading to irreversible lens cell damage.

The types of cataract are shown in Figure 4.1.

Cortical cataract formation is the most frequent with typical radial spoke-like opacities. Nuclear and subcapsular (anterior or posterior) cataracts may result in reduction and blurring of vision, as well as problems with the headlights of oncoming cars and bright sunlight. True diabetic cataracts are a result of osmotic overhydration of the lens and appear as bilateral white snowflake opacities, which may mature over days.

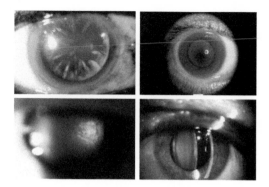

Figure 4.1 **Types of cataracts.** Top left, cortical cataract; top right, white complete lens opacity. Bottom left, posterior subcapsular lens opacity; bottom right, nuclear lens opacity.

Reproduced courtesy of Professor Paul M. Dodson and The Heart of England Retinal Screening Centre.

## 4.3 Retinovascular disease

Retinovascular disease is more common in diabetic subjects, largely due to the excess of cardiovascular risk factors in diabetics, which are involved in the aetiology. Examples of retinal occlusion are shown in Figure 4.2.

The aetiology of retinal vein occlusion (RVO) is multifactorial, but the primary event is damage to the wall of the venous vasculature. The major risk factors are hypertension and hyperlipidaemia, which are strongly associated with diabetes. In the diabetic retinopathy screening programme (DESP), RVO less commonly presents with a fresh acute appearance and more commonly with features of a previous old RVO that may include residual haemorrhage, ghost vessels, collateral vessel formation, and sector retinal laser scars.

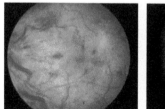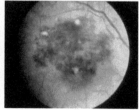

Figure 4.2 **Retinal vein occlusion.** Left panel shows a central retinal vein occlusion and the right panel, the branch form.

Reproduced courtesy of Professor Paul M. Dodson and The Heart of England Retinal Screening Centre.

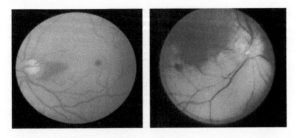

Figure 4.3 Retinal arteriolar occlusion. Left panel shows an acute central retinal artery occlusion and the right panel a branch retinal artery occlusion due to a cholesterol embolus blocking the inferior temporal artery.

Reproduced courtesy of Professor Paul M. Dodson and The Heart of England Retinal Screening Centre.

Retinal artery occlusion (RAO) occurs in both the central and branch form, although it is less common than RVO. RAO relates to the same risk factors as RVO, but is also strongly related to cigarette smoking. It is very rare to see fresh RAO on screening photographs, but more commonly old retinal changes, including ghost vessels and those of pale thinned retina.

Examples of retinal artery occlusion are shown in Figure 4.3.

Non-arteritic ischaemic optic neuropathy occurs when there is occlusion to the posterior ciliary artery supply to the optic nerve, resulting in painless visual loss in the form of an altitudinal field defect. The retinal appearance is shown in Figure 4.4. The risk factors are similar to retinal artery occlusion.

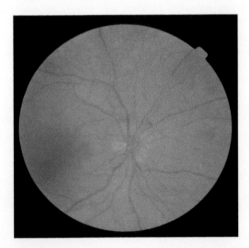

Figure 4.4 Ischaemic optic neuropathy with swelling of the optic nerve head.

Reproduced courtesy of Professor Paul M. Dodson and The Heart of England Retinal Screening Centre.

Retinovascular disease is an important cause of visual loss in diabetic subjects, such that medical investigation and tight control of cardiovascular risk factors should help in prevention, as well as recurrence in the fellow eye with potential disastrous visual outcome.

## 4.4 Glaucoma

Primary open angle glaucoma (POAG) is increased in the diabetic population. This may lead to visual loss due to progressive loss of optic nerve fibres. This is due to direct injury due to raised intra-ocular pressure or progressive infarction of the microcirculation of the optic nerve head. The typical sign of classic glaucoma is cupping of the optic disc (see Figure 4.5).

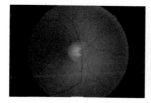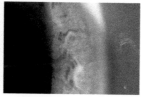

Figure 4.5 Cupping of the optic disc (left panel) and new vessels on the surface of the iris, termed iris rubeosis or iris neovascularization (right panel).
Reproduced courtesy of Professor Paul M. Dodson and The Heart of England Retinal Screening Centre.

Glaucoma may also be due to advanced diabetic eye disease with new vessels growing on the iris (Figure 4.5) termed iris neovascularization (iris rubeosis). The neovascularization of the iris obstructs the drainage angle of the eye (the canal of Schlemm), and is accompanied by fibrosis leading to rubeotic glaucoma and extremely high intra-ocular pressure. The optic nerve rapidly atrophies and the eye may become rapidly painful.

## 4.5 Cranial nerve palsies

Neuropathy of the third, fourth, and sixth cranial nerves may result in extra-ocular muscle palsies, which may be the presentation of undiagnosed diabetes mellitus. These present with double vision (diplopia), usually painless, and will slowly resolve within 6 months of onset. The pathology is segmental demyelination of the affected nerve secondary to ischaemia produced by microangiopathy (small vessel disease).

## 4.6 Diabetic retinopathy

Diabetic small vessel disease (diabetic microangiopathy) is a specific, but at the same time generalized, disorder of small blood vessels. It is specific in that it only occurs in patients with diabetes, but generalized in that it can appear in virtually every small vessel in the body. The histological hallmark of microangiopathy is capillary basement membrane thickening. In addition, the basement membrane architecture becomes abnormal and porous, causing leakage of plasma protein that, in turn, leads to the development of profound abnormalities within the microcirculation. The principal vascular beds that are affected include the eyes (retinopathy), the kidneys (nephropathy), and the neurovascular bundle of peripheral nerves (neuropathy).

Hyperglycaemia affects retinal blood flow and metabolism, and has a direct effect on the cells associated with retinal circulation. There is loss of retinal pericytes in the capillary walls, which are needed to maintain retinal vascular autoregulation of blood flow and the endothelial cell lining.

The pathogenetic role of hyperglycaemia is proven, although it is not known precisely how glucose toxicity results in retinopathy, but there are a number of potential effects on the retinal perfusion and metabolic pathways, which result in vascular leakage and retinal ischaemia shown in Figure 4.6. A stained histological preparation of a retina with diabetic changes is shown in Figure 4.7, demonstrating the formation of microaneurysms and capillary closure. An exact description of the stages of DR is given in detail in later chapters.

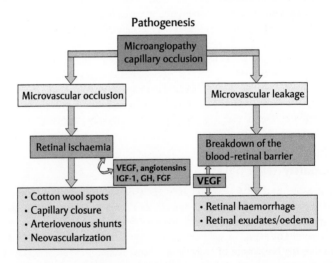

**Figure 4.6** An illustration of the changes that occur in the development of diabetic retinopathy (DR) and pathogenetic factors.

VEGF, vascular endothelial growth factor; IGF-1, insulin-like growth factor 1; GH, growth hormone; FGF, fibroblast growth factor.

Reproduced courtesy of Professor Paul M. Dodson and The Heart of England Retinal Screening Centre.

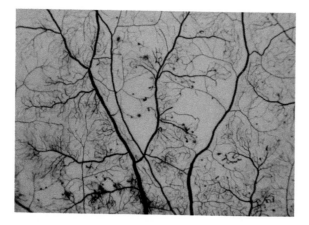

Figure 4.7 A stain of a retinal section outlining the vasculature and key changes in DR. Retinal capillaries have been outlined and demonstrate the changes of microaneurysms and areas of capillary non-perfusion.

The consequences of hyperglycaemia include capillary cell death, alteration of retinal pericyte/endothelial cell ratio, and vascular occlusion. Increased blood flow in the capillaries occurs due to loss of pericytes in the normal retina, leading to disruption of retinal blood flow autoregulation. The resulting increased blood flow affects the capillary wall by stimulating production of vaso-active substances and increasing endothelial cell proliferation, eventually resulting in the closure of the capillary circulation. This leads to a state of chronic hypoxia (low oxygen) in the retina and increases in the levels of a number of growth factors, including vascular endothelial growth factor (VEGF), insulin-like growth factor 1 (IGF-1), and fibroblast growth factor (FGF).

## 4.7 Epidemiology and risk factors for diabetic retinopathy

DR is one of the most common causes of blindness in the working population of the developed world and a significant cause of blindness in the elderly population.

The risk of DR increases with disease duration. Epidemiological studies have shown that the prevalence of DR is greater than 95% after 15 years of disease in patients diagnosed with diabetes before the age of 30 (principally Type 1 diabetes). Of those diagnosed after that age, 20% have signs of retinopathy at diagnosis, rising to 60% after 15 years of Type 2 diabetes. In the UK, around 30–35% of all patients with diabetes have DR, 1–2% are partially sighted or blind, and approximately 300 new cases of blindness are registered every year.

Recent data from the digital camera DESP have demonstrated more accurate prevalence rates, with ~30–35% of all diabetics having some form of DR and 3–5% with sight-threatening maculopathy.

Ethnic differences are apparent with an increased rate of retinopathy and maculopathy in diabetic patients of Asian or Afro-Caribbean origin, as shown in Figure 4.8.

There are differences between the two types of diabetes. In Type 1 diabetes, DR is almost invariable with greater than 95% affected after 15 years duration. In contrast, 20% have signs of DR at diagnosis of Type 2 diabetes, rising to 60% after 15 years known duration (see Figure 4.9).

In children with Type 1 diabetes, it is rare to observe DR before 6 years of diabetes duration, such that the youngest diabetic patient reported with sight-threatening DR in the literature is older than 11 years of age. While there is an increased prevalence related to puberty, the recommended age to start screening for DR has therefore been set to >12 years. However, diabetes is now presenting in babies and, therefore, individual decisions will need to be made as to when to start screening (for example, age at diabetes diagnosis plus 6 years).

With regard to type of DR, 50% of patients with Type 1 diabetes and approximately 10% of those with Type 2 diabetes will have proliferative DR after 15 years known duration of the disease. While around 5% of patients in cross-sectional studies will need to be referred for ophthalmological examination because of sight-threatening maculopathy, the incidence of macular oedema over a period of 10 years is 20% in Type 1 diabetic subjects, and 25% in Type 2 patients requiring insulin, versus 13.9% in Type 2 diabetic patients who did not. The latter reinforces the importance of insulin therapy as shown in Figure 4.10. This also demonstrates the crucial role of increasing duration of diabetes in the development of DR.

|                      | Established (A) | New digital (B) | Asian (C) |
|----------------------|-----------------|-----------------|-----------|
| Normal (R0)          | 57%             | 47%             | 54.4%     |
| Maculopathy (M1)     | 5%              | 7.5%            | 12.7%     |
| Preproliferative (R2)| 3%              | 1.1%            | 1%        |
| Proliferative (R3)   | 1%              | 1.2%            | 3%        |
| Referral rate        | 7.8%            | 10%             | 16.4%     |
| Ungradable           | 1.8%            | 2%              | –         |

Figure 4.8 Prevalence rates of DR and referral rates for a well-established digital camera screened diabetic population (A), a newly digitally screened population (B) in South Birmingham, and from the UK Asian study (C) in Birmingham and Coventry.

The R system (R0, R1, R2, R3) are the retinopathy levels used in the English Diabetic Retinopathy Screening Programme (see Chapter 11, 'How to grade').

Reproduced courtesy of Professor Paul M. Dodson and The Heart of England Retinal Screening Centre.

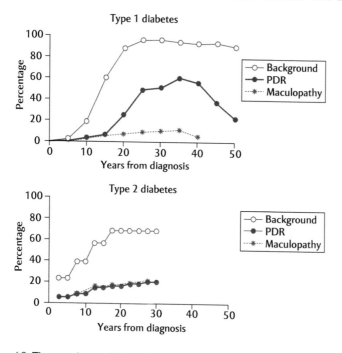

Figure 4.9 The prevalence of DR in Type 1 and Type 2 diabetes demonstrating the tight relationship with increasing duration in both types.

PDR, proliferative diabetic retinopathy.

Reproduced courtesy of Professor Paul M. Dodson and The Heart of England Retinal Screening Centre.

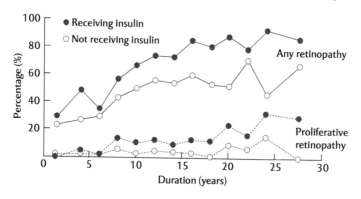

Figure 4.10 The prevalence of DR (%) in those on insulin compared with those not on insulin and the relationship to duration of diabetes.

Reproduced courtesy of Professor Paul M. Dodson and The Heart of England Retinal Screening Centre.

Note that, in general;

- Proliferative retinopathy is more common in Type 1 diabetes.
- Maculopathy is more strongly associated with Type 2 diabetes.
- 80% of cases registered visually impaired or blind due to DR are due to diabetic maculopathy.
- Modern management of Type 1 diabetes and appropriate ophthalmological care, including timely vitrectomy surgery, have resulted in blindness being relatively rare due to proliferative retinopathy.

### 4.7.1 Risk factors for development of diabetic retinopathy

The risk factors for development of DR are:

- increasing duration of diabetes mellitus;
- type of diabetes (more common in Type 1 diabetes than Type 2);
- increased blood pressure (BP);
- poor glycaemic control;
- presence of macro- or micro-albuminuria;
- increasing serum cholesterol levels;
- pregnancy;
- cigarette smoking;
- obstructive sleep apnoea.

The first two risk factors listed of increased duration and type of diabetes are non-modifiable risk factors, but the others listed are modifiable, and medical management is aimed at optimizing glycaemic and BP control, with attention to lipid levels and cessation of cigarette smoking as outlined in Chapter 1, 'What is diabetes?', and Chapter 16, 'Medical management of diabetic retinopathy'.

Epidemiological studies have also confirmed that increasing serum cholesterol and triglyceride levels are related to the development of macular exudation, macular oedema, and proliferative retinopathy, see Figure 4.11.

The presence of micro- or macro-albuminuria is a strong predictor of DR, not surprising in that it, too, is a microvascular complication with similar risk factors, but is also common in both Types 1 and 2 diabetics.

Diabetic pregnancy is a definite risk factor for increased progression of DR, as reports have shown that DR may progress very rapidly with visual loss during pregnancy. The predictive factors for deterioration include the presence of proteinuria and pre-existing retinopathy changes before pregnancy (see chapter 17).

The relationship between smoking and retinopathy is unclear, as some studies have shown smoking to be an adverse factor, while others have almost suggested cigarette smoking to be protective.

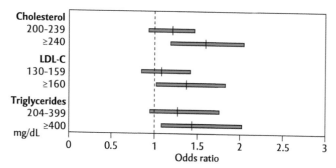

**Figure 4.11** Relationship of serum lipids to retinal exudation from the ETDRS study.

Note: Controlling for other independent risk factors in multiple logistic regression models. ETDRS, Early Treatment Diabetic Retinopathy Study. LDL-C, low density lipoprotein cholesterol.

Reproduced courtesy of Professor Paul M. Dodson and The Heart of England Retinal Screening Centre.

While genetic influences may have a role in diabetic nephropathy, there is some weak evidence to suggest that there could be a genetic component. Familial clustering of severe vision-threatening DR was observed in the Diabetes Control and Complications Trial (DCCT), and the continued progression of DR after institution of normoglycaemia may be consistent with altered critical gene expression induced by chronic hyperglycaemia.

Special circumstances are relevant to clinical care. It is well established that DR may deteriorate with a rapid and major improvement in glycaemic control. This commonly follows the institution of insulin therapy, leading to more frequent retinal examination. Although the mechanism of the deterioration is not clear, there is a benefit of improved glycaemic control in the longer term. Patients with diabetic nephropathy also have a higher risk of deterioration, such that patients either approaching dialysis or with a low glomerular filtration rate (GFR) should be more frequently monitored.

## FURTHER READING

Beri MR, Klugman MR, Kohler JA, Hayreh SS. (1987). Anterior ischaemic optic neuropathy. VII. Incidence of bilaterality and various influencing factors. *Ophthalmology* **94**: 1020–8.

Broadbent DM, Scott JA, Vora JP, Harding SP. (1999). Prevalence of diabetic eye disease in an inner city population: the Liverpool Diabetic Eye Study. *Eye* **13**: 160–5.

Chowdhury TA, Hopkins D, Dodson PM, Vafidis GC. (2002). The role of serum lipids in exudative diabetic maculopathy: is there a place for lipid lowering therapy? *Eye* **16**: 689–93.

Dodson PM, Gibson JM, Kritzinger EE. (1995). Retinal artery occlusion. In: Allen C, Ho MD (eds) *Clinical retinopathies*, pp. 77–83. Chapman and Hall, London.

Dodson PM, Gibson JM, Kritzinger EE. (1995). Retinal vein occlusion. In: Allen C, Ho MD (eds) *Clinical retinopathies*, pp. 85–93. Chapman and Hall, London.

Donaldson M, Dodson PM. (2003). Medical treatment of diabetic retinopathy. *Eye* **17**: 550–62.

Frank RN. (2004). Diabetic retinopathy. *N Engl J Med* **350**: 48–58.

Gale R, Scanlon PH, Evans M, Ghanchi F, Yang Y, Silvestri G, et al. (2017). Action on diabetic macular oedema: achieving optimal patient management in treating visual impairment due to diabetic eye disease. *Eye* **31**: S1–S20.

Klein R, Klein BE, Moss SE, Davis MD, DeMets DL. (1984). The Wisconsin Epidemiologic study of diabetic retinopathy: III. The prevalence and risk of diabetic retinopathy when age at diagnosis is 30 years or more years. *Arch Ophthalmol* **102**: 527–32.

Klein R, Klein BE, Scot E, Moss SE, Cruickshanks K. (1998). The Wisconsin Epidemiologic Study of Diabetic Retinopathy: XVII. The 14-year incidence and progression of diabetic retinopathy and associated risk factors in type 1 diabetes. *Ophthalmology* **105**: 1801–15.

Klein B, Moss SE, Klein R. (1990). The effect of pregnancy on the progression of diabetic retinopathy. *Diabetes Care* **13**: 34.

Prasad S, Kamath GG, Jones K, Clearkin LG, Phillips RP. (2001). Prevalence of blindness and visual impairment in a population of people with diabetes. *Eye* **15**: 640–3.

Royal College of Ophthalmology—Diabetic Retinopathy Guidelines—DR Guidelines Expert Working Party. www.rcophth.ac.uk (accessed 8 August 2019).

Schmidt-Erfurth U, Garcia-Arumi J, Bandello F, Berg K, Chakravarthy U, Gerendas BS, et al. (2017). Guidelines for the management of diabetic macula oedema by the European Society of retina Specialists (EURETINA). *Ophthalmologica* **237**: 185–222.

Wong TY, Sun J, Kawasaki R, Ruamviboonsuk P, Gupta N, Lansingh VC, et al. (2018). Guidelines on diabetic eye care: The International Council of Ophthalmology recommendations for screening, follow-up, referral, and treatment based on resource settings. *Ophthalmology* **125**(10): 1608–22.

# Background diabetic retinopathy

Rachel Stockwin and Emma Shepherd

**KEY POINTS**

- Background changes are, as their name suggests, not visually threatening.
- Background changes, if identified for the first time, are a warning sign that microvascular disease is present.
- Background changes are common, affecting up to 40% of the diabetic population.
- Background diabetic retinopathy (DR) consists of:
  - microaneurysms;
  - haemorrhages;
  - exudates;
  - cotton wool spots;
  - venous loops.

## 5.1 Background diabetic retinopathy

Background DR is the term used for DR in its earliest and least sight-threatening forms. It is either less developed than other referable stages of retinopathy, or found further away from the fovea and, therefore, is less of a threat to central vision.

Background DR does not, in itself, disrupt visual function. The presence of any of the main features—microaneurysms, haemorrhages, exudate, cotton wool spots, or venous loops—does indicate, however, a susceptibility to further retinal damage. A referral to ophthalmology may not be necessary at this stage, but attention to blood glucose and blood pressure (BP) control is important.

## 5.2 Microaneurysms

Microaneurysms (see Figure 5.1) are commonly found in the early stages of DR. Weakening of the capillary wall causes swelling and small red dots become

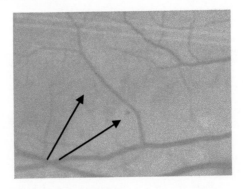

Figure 5.1 **Microaneurysms (arrowed).**
Reproduced courtesy of Professor Paul M. Dodson and The Heart of England Retinal Screening Centre.

visible in the retina. These may be few and far between, or widespread across the fundus. Microaneurysms are usually clearly identifiable, although they can be similar in appearance to the ends of vessels (vessels rising up through the retinal vasculature, rather than along the retina) or colour variations of a healthy fundus. They are usually found clear of the main vessels and distinct in appearance.

On their own, microaneurysms constitute little threat to vision. If, however, there is a non-historical or sudden reduction in visual acuity to 6/12 (0.3 LogMAR), or worse, and microaneurysms are present near the fovea, then this ceases to be background retinopathy and a referral to ophthalmology for maculopathy may be necessary (see Chapter 6, 'Maculopathy').

## 5.3 Haemorrhages

Haemorrhages are commonly seen in DR, although some have other causes such as the valsalva effect (a rise in pressure of the chest cavity, leading to a rise in venous pressure, due to straining, such as in coughing, sneezing, or constipation) or systemic blood disorders (such as anaemia or leukaemia). In background DR, intra-retinal haemorrhages originate from ruptured capillaries within the retina. These capillaries are deeper than those with microaneurysms and the circumference of a haemorrhage is usually greater as a result. Haemorrhages are approximately round in appearance (dot or blot appearance) and appear in the deeper layers of the retina (the inner nuclear and outer plexiform layers) (see Figure 5.2). As with the other main forms of background DR, the haemorrhages themselves do not disturb visual function.

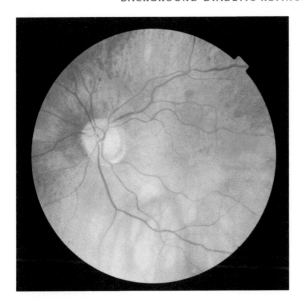

Figure 5.2 **Haemorrhages and Microaneurysms.**

Both haemorrhages and microaneurysms can deteriorate, needing treatment, or they can resolve over time. In conjunction with a visual acuity of 6/12 (0.3 LogMAR) or worse, haemorrhages can require referral for maculopathy if within 1 disc diameter of the fovea.

## 5.4 Exudation

Abnormalities in the lining of the capillary can lead to leakage of the lipoproteins in the blood into surrounding tissues, resulting in lipid or fat deposition in the retina, and referred to as exudation, with a yellow, waxy appearance. This usually occurs in the presence of other features of DR. This, combined with their well-defined edges, helps to differentiate them from other retinal pigment epithelium changes or reflective particles. Exudate may appear in a variety of patterns, including individual patches, tracking lines, part of a circle (termed circinates) and, if in the macula, macula star appearance. Formations of exudate that occur in the macular region are therefore considered to be maculopathy (see Figure 5.3), as opposed to background DR (see Chapter 6, 'Maculopathy'). Outside the macula, exudates are most commonly seen in small patches, clumps, and circinates.

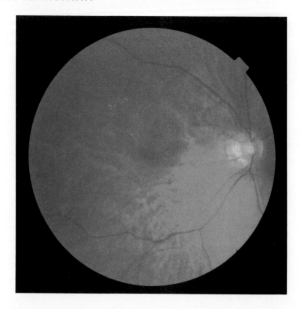

Figure 5.3 Exudate forming circinate and tracking into the fovea, thereby comprising maculopathy.

## 5.5 Cotton wool spots

Cotton wool spots are ischaemic lesions in the nerve fibre layer of the retina (see Figure 5.4). They are caused by a localized failure of the capillary network to feed and provide oxygen. Cotton wool spots have a characteristic fluffy, white

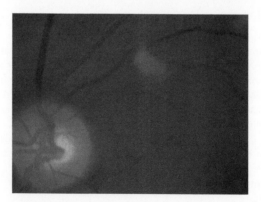

Figure 5.4 Cotton wool spot.

Reproduced courtesy of Professor Paul M. Dodson and The Heart of England Retinal Screening Centre.

appearance (hence their name), which fades over time. In digital photography, this fluffy appearance generally makes them clearly identifiable, although they may occasionally resemble retinal pigment epithelium (RPE) change or camera artefacts.

Cotton wool spots may occur with other features of DR, such as microaneurysms and haemorrhages. Care needs to be taken when screening, to ensure that features of pre-proliferative retinopathy are not present (see Chapter 7, 'Pre-proliferative and proliferative retinopathy'). A number of other conditions also cause cotton wool spots, notably hypertension, pregnancy, and the contraceptive pill. Due to this, cotton wool spots alone are not classed as background DR.

## 5.6 Venous loops

Venous loops are abnormalities that are usually noticed on large retinal veins (see Figure 5.5). Changes in vessel walls leading to weakening can alter the camber of vessels. This appears as a bend or loop in the vein or artery. These do not constitute DR alone, but are relevant when combined with other pathologies.

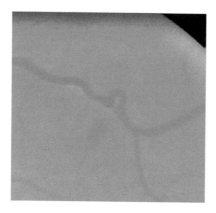

Figure 5.5 **Venous loop.**

## 5.7 Summary

Background DR is not, in itself, sight-threatening. It is a good indicator that the retina is not healthy, but is at a stage when annual recall for screening is still the best outcome of the screening event (the same outcome as if no retinopathy is present). Many of the same features, such as microaneurysms, haemorrhages, and cotton wool spots can constitute referable retinopathy in different circumstances (see Chapter 6, 'Maculopathy', and Chapter 7, 'Pre-proliferative and proliferative retinopathy') and, with this in mind, screeners should have a clear grasp of why the pathology discovered is classified as background, and what can change a grade from background retinopathy to maculopathy or pre-proliferative DR.

## FURTHER READING

Butcher A, Dodson PM. (2001). In: Sinclair AJ, Finucane P (eds) *Diabetes in Old Age*. John Wiley and Sons Ltd, Oxford.

Dodson PM, Gibson JM, Kritzinger EE. (1995). In: *Clinical retinopathies*. Chapman and Hall, London.

CHAPTER 5

# CHAPTER 6

# Maculopathy

Helen Wharton

---

**KEY POINTS**

- This chapter will examine the physiological changes within the macula that can lead to diabetic macular oedema (DMO), how these are detected at diabetic eye screening (DES), and the consequences this has on patient management.
- It will look at how the area of the macula is defined on the fundus image and the different surrogate markers used during screening to predict the presence of DMO. The grading criteria for maculopathy (M1) as defined by the NHS Diabetic Eye Screening Programme (NHSDESP) are described, which includes single exudates, groups of exudates, and haemorrhages and microaneurysms with reduced visual acuity (VA).
- It will examine the classification of different maculopathies, such as exudative (focal and diffuse), cystoid, and ischaemic, and includes images of their appearance on retinal images.
- Management of patients with maculopathy, such as referral to the hospital eye service (HES) or digital surveillance (DS) clinics, and treatment of DMO, including laser and intra-vitreal injections, will also be briefly mentioned.

---

## 6.1 Introduction to diabetic maculopathy

Diabetic maculopathy is the commonest cause of blindness in people with diabetes. It results from a build-up of fluid called oedema in the macula area of the retina. If oedema occurs in the central part of the macula, this is called central involving diabetic macular oedema (CIDMO), which carries a high risk of loss of central vision. Approximately 7% of people with diabetes in the United Kingdom have diabetic maculopathy, of whom 39% have CIDMO. The prevalence of maculopathy increases with diabetes duration and severity, as well as other risk factors, such as hypertension and increased cholesterol levels. Various studies have shown a direct relationship between maculopathy and vision, indicating a decrease in visual acuity with increasing severity of diabetic maculopathy. This emphasizes the importance of screening for diabetic maculopathy, as it is an asymptomatic disease in the earlier stages of development. Treatment is most effective at this stage as it is more likely to result in a better visual outcome.

### 6.1.1 Anatomical features of the macula

According to current NHSDESP criteria, the macula is defined as the area of the retina that lies within a circle centred on the fovea, whose radius is the distance between the temporal margin of the disc and the centre of the fovea (Figure 6.1). The macula is highly sensitive and is primarily responsible for central vision. Within the centre of the macula lies a pit known as the fovea. The fovea is the thinnest part of the retina and consists of a high concentration of cone cells, which are responsible for central vision, fine visual acuity, and colour vision (see Chapter 3, 'Anatomy of the eye and the healthy fundus'). Diabetic changes, such as microaneurysms, exudates, or oedema in this area will probably be sight threatening due to disruption of the arrangement of photoreceptors. This can affect central visual acuity, resulting in blurring of vision and is recorded on visual acuity testing.

### 6.1.2 Development of diabetic maculopathy

Diabetes can alter the physical properties of the retinal vasculature, which may result in maculopathy. Changes in blood flow due to hyperglycaemia lead to vascular changes within the small vessels, resulting in vascular abnormalities that disrupt vascular flow. As the basement membrane thickens, this causes the loss of pericytes from retinal vessel walls. Pericytes are contractile cells that control vascular blood flow via autoregulation. The loss of control increases the blood flow and pressure within the vessel lumen, leading to the loss of tight junctions in the endothelial wall, which maintain the blood–retinal barrier, hence increasing blood flow and capillary permeability. Changes in the vascular structure of the vessel endothelium and blood flow leads to the capillary leakage of blood, lipids, protein, and water. The breakdown of the endothelial wall leads to the early clinical signs seen in diabetic maculopathy, such as exudates and macular oedema (exudative maculopathy). Capillary closure will also occur at an advanced stage

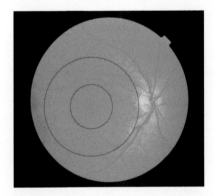

Figure 6.1 Anatomical area of the macula. The inner circle indicates 1DD from the centre of the fovea and the outer circle indicates the whole macula region.

due to increased perfusion pressure at the capillaries, causing infiltration of cells, and swelling, which causes blockage and resultant macula ischaemia (ischaemic maculopathy).

## 6.1.3 Screening for diabetic maculopathy

Macular oedema and retinal thickening is difficult to distinguish on a flat two-dimensional (2D) image. Positive identification of these features requires a three-dimensional (3D) view, such as that performed by slit lamp biomicroscopy examination or optical coherence tomography (OCT). As flat 2D digital images are used during screening, it is therefore necessary to identify macula changes that can be identified on a 2D view that strongly correlate and predict the presence of macular oedema at a stage where treatment will result in the best visual outcome. These are called surrogate markers. Following a literature review, a grading committee advised on a list of retinal changes to be the best surrogate markers for macular oedema. This list was updated in 2012 by the NHSDESP and forms part of the grading criteria for referable retinopathy. NHSDESP stipulated that the best surrogate markers for predicting the presence of macular oedema and, hence, referable maculopathy includes:

- exudate within one disc diameter (1DD) of the centre of the fovea;
- a group of exudates within the macula, greater than or equal to half the disc area;
- retinal thickening within 1DD of the fovea (if stereo available);
- any microaneurysm or haemorrhage within 1DD of the centre of the fovea with best corrected visual acuity of 6/12 (0.3 LogMAR) or worse.

In summary, the surrogate markers stipulated by the NHSDESP are used as the definition of referable maculopathy, which is termed maculopathy (M1) and should be appropriately managed by close monitoring or treatment. Patients with early macula changes will usually be asymptomatic, thus stressing the importance of regular and accurate DES.

## 6.2 Classification of diabetic maculopathies

Maculopathy can occur in stages from early maculopathy to end-stage oedematous maculopathy. The three main types of diabetic maculopathy are exudative (focal or diffuse), ischaemic, and cystoid. A mixed form of exudative and ischaemic maculopathies is also common.

### 6.2.1 Early maculopathy

The use of grading software allows for enhancement and magnification of the retinal images to identify the very early signs of maculopathy. A visual acuity (VA) of

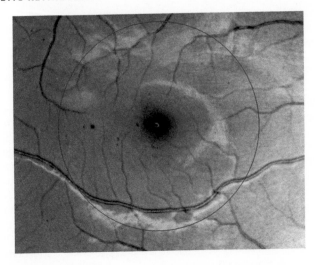

Figure 6.2 Early maculopathy. Clinical features of small microaneurysms located within 1DD of the fovea shown in red-free.

6/12 (0.3 LogMAR) or worse (especially where there has been a reduction in VA) accompanied by microaneurysm or haemorrhage within 1DD of the fovea may indicate early signs of significant maculopathy and should be graded M1 (Figure 6.2). However, in cases where poor VA is not thought to be due to maculopathy, for example, due to amblyopia or other conditions, such as age-related macular degeneration (AMD) or cataracts, then an appropriate clinical decision on outcome should be made.

### 6.2.2 Exudative maculopathy

Exudative maculopathy occurs due to the release of lipoproteins and water from retinal capillaries. It is characterized by thick, yellow, waxy deposits of exudates with sharp defined borders. These types of retinal exudates tend to accumulate in the outer plexiform layer. They may appear as discrete singular flecks of exudates within 1DD of the fovea (Figure 6.3), or may occur in groups and form certain patterns. Exudates within the macula may begin to encroach on the fovea; these exudates are derived from vessels in the macula area and are located between the radially arranged fibres of Henle's layer. This type of exudation is known as tracking (Figure 6.4) and may cause deterioration in vision if it starts to impinge on the fovea. Any exudates within 1DD of the fovea should be graded as M1.

Exudative maculopathy is further subdivided into focal and diffuse maculopathy, which are characterized by the area of exudate and oedema within the macula.

Figure 6.3 Single exudate leakage within 1DD.

### 6.2.2.1 *Focal maculopathy (non-central involving diabetic macular oedema)*

Focal maculopathy is characterized by the distribution of exudates throughout the posterior pole. Exudates may occur in a group or take on a flattened ring-like shape called a circinate (Figure 6.4). In a circinate, the finely defined thick, yellow deposits of lipid leakage can form around a retinal microaneurysm or capillary leakage. Focal exudation is usually localized to one part of the macula region and is more commonly seen in the temporal area of the macula, known as the

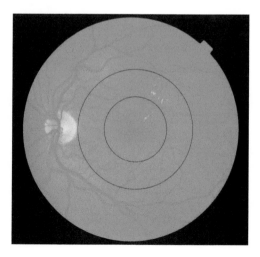

Figure 6.4 Tracking exudate within 1DD and a circinate greater than half the area of the optic disc within the macula area.

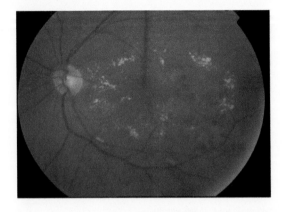

Figure 6.5 Diffuse maculopathy (CIDMO). Characteristic appearance of diffuse oedema and exudation affecting the whole macula region.
Reproduced courtesy of Professor Paul M. Dodson and The Heart of England Retinal Screening Centre.

watershed area. If a group of exudates or circinate is equivalent to or greater in size to half the area of the optic disc (OD) and is all within the macula then this should be graded as M1. To determine the size of a group, an imaginary line can be drawn around the outer exudates and the area of this can be compared to half the OD.

Vision only becomes affected when the exudates begin to encroach upon the fovea. If macular oedema is significant in this area it may be treated by focal macula laser surgery (see Chapter 19, 'Ophthalmic treatment of diabetic retinopathy').

### 6.2.2.2 Diffuse maculopathy (central involving diabetic macular oedema)

Diffuse maculopathy occurs when exudates surround the whole macula (Figure 6.5). It is usually more advanced than focal maculopathy and the generalized thickening of the macula is associated with deterioration in vision. Grid laser may be used to treat this type of maculopathy, but the response to laser is more limited so anti-vascular endothelial growth factor (VEGF) injection therapy or corticosteroids has become the treatment of choice (see Chapter 20, 'New treatment strategies for diabetic eye disease').

### 6.2.3 Ischaemic maculopathy

Ischaemic maculopathy occurs due to hypoperfusion (retinal capillary closure) of the macula and requires urgent ophthalmology referral. It is characterized by a pale macula (due to deprived retinal circulation) accompanied by blot haemorrhages, macular oedema, and cotton wool spots (Figure 6.6). Further

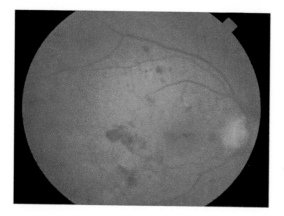

Figure 6.6 Ischaemic maculopathy. A distinctive fundus image of ischaemic maculopathy showing a pale macula and large blot haemorrhages.

Reproduced courtesy of Professor Paul M. Dodson and The Heart of England Retinal Screening Centre.

investigations of retinal leakage/oedema are detected by fundus fluorescein angiograms, slit lamp biomicroscopy or OCT, which highlights areas of retinal thickening and ischaemia (see Chapter 18, 'Imaging in Diabetic Retinopathy', under the chapter headings fundus fluorescein angiography(FFA), optical coherence tomography (OCT), and optical coherence tomography angiography (OCTA)). A clinician may decide that a patient with ischaemic maculopathy needs to be seen soon in the HES, as this type of maculopathy poses a significant risk to vision because it is less responsive to treatment and focal laser treatment is contraindicated.

### 6.2.4 Cystoid maculopathy

Cystoid maculopathy occurs due to accumulation of extracellular fluid from the retinal capillaries into the macula area, causing retinal thickening. This indicates a breakdown of the inner blood–retinal barrier. It is characterized by a significant reduction in central vision and multiple petals around the macula, representing cysts full of fluid (Figure 6.7). Cystoid changes associated with diffuse or focal maculopathy frequently have a poorer prognosis and a disappointing response to treatment, which can lead to irreversible loss of vision.

## 6.3 Management of diabetic maculopathy

There are two possible outcomes for screen positive M1. These are either referral to a DS clinic for close monitoring or referral to the HES for monitoring or treatment.

Figure 6.7 Cystoid maculopathy. Clinical features of multiple petals pattern around the macula representing localized macular oedema.
Reproduced courtesy of Professor Paul M. Dodson and The Heart of England Retinal Screening Centre.

Since OCT is an integral part in the diagnosis and management of maculopathy it has become increasingly popular in DS to help identify those patients who require a true referral to HES, thereby reducing the burden of patients into ophthalmology clinics (see Chapter 17, 'Patients of concern'). It has been found that only around 20% of patients with features of M1 at screening will have macular oedema. This shows that the majority of patients with M1 do not require treatment and can be managed in DS clinics. A recent article by Scanlon (2018) has suggested a consensus grading criteria for macular OCT findings in patients with M1 to provide guidance and standardization, if outcomes are being decided by technicians.

Current guidelines set by NHSDESP for M1 referrals are:

- To HES, a minimum of 70% of patients should be seen within 13 weeks from the date of screening.
- To DS, a minimum of 70% should be seen within 3 months from the date of screening.

## 6.4  Summary

Maculopathy is the largest cause of blindness due to diabetic retinopathy. It is therefore essential that regular and accurate DES is in place to detect surrogate markers, which can identify early asymptomatic DMO. Early and timely treatment can be applied if needed, thereby preventing avoidable vision loss. The different types and features of maculopathy are summarized in Table 6.1.

**Table 6.1** Classification of diabetic maculopathy

| Types of macula disease | Clinical features | Diabetic maculopathy grade | Outcome |
|---|---|---|---|
| Exudative (focal) | Exudates concentrated in one area of the macula | M1 | Referral to HES |
| Exudative (diffuse) | Exudates surrounding the macula | M1 | Referral to HES |
| Ischaemic maculopathy | Pale macula, cotton wool spots, and blot haemorrhages | M1 | Referral to HES |
| Cystoid maculopathy | Retinal thickening and characteristic petals | M1 | Referral to HES |

FURTHER READING

Brownlee M. (2001). Biochemistry and molecular cell biology of diabetic complications. *Nature* **414**(6865): 813–20.

Cook HL, Newsom R, Long V, Smith SA, Shilling JS, Stanford MR. (1999). Natural history of diabetic macular streak exudates: evidence from a screening programme. *Br J Ophthalmol* **83**: 563–6.

Dodson PM, Gibson JM, Kritzinger EE. (1995). *Clinical Retinopathies*. Chapman and Hall Medical, Abingdon.

NICE. (2015). Aflibercept for treating diabetic macular oedema—guidance, Technology appraisal guideline TA346. https://www.nice.org.uk/guidance/ta346 (accessed 9 August 2019).

Prescott G, Sharp P, Goatman K, Scotland G, Fleming A, et al. (2014). Improving the cost-effectiveness of photographic screening for diabetic macular oedema: a prospective, multi-centre, UK study. *Br J Ophthalmol* **98**(8): 1042–9.

Public Health England. (2017). NHS Diabetic Eye Screening Programme; grading definitions for referable disease. Public Health England, London.

Scanlon P. (2018). Digital surveillance with OCT and the treatment of diabetic macular oedema. *Diabetic Eye J* **11**: 6–11.

Wharton HM, Gibson JM, Dodson PM. (2011). How accurate are photographic surrogate markers used to detect macular oedema in the English National Screening Programme? *Eur J Ophthalmol* **21**(3): 343–52.

Zander E, Herfurth S, Bohl B, Heinke P, Herrmann U, Kohnert KD, et al. (2000). Maculopathy in patients with diabetes mellitus type 1 and type 2: associations with risk factors. *Br J Ophthalmol* **84**: 871–6.

# CHAPTER 7

# Pre-proliferative and proliferative retinopathy

Prashant Amrelia

---

**KEY POINTS**

- Pre-proliferative retinopathy precedes proliferative retinopathy (new vessel growth) and, therefore, is an indication that the eye will soon be moving on to the advanced stages of retinopathy.
- Pre-proliferative retinopathy indicates chronic retinal ischaemia, due to blocked capillaries and the clinical sign/s that include:
  - multiple deep round blot haemorrhages;
  - intra-retinal microvascular abnormalities (IRMA);
  - venous beading;
  - venous reduplication.
- New vessels at the optic disc (NVD) or new vessels elsewhere (NVE) on the retinal surface arise due to retinal ischaemia and increased vascular endothelial growth factor (VEGF) and others factors.
- The new vessels help compensate the hypoxic (oxygen-starved) tissue. These new vessels can easily rupture, leading to haemorrhage (vitreous haemorrhage) and severe visual loss.

---

## 7.1 Pre-proliferative retinopathy

Pre-proliferative retinopathy is a clinically identifiable stage of diabetic retinopathy (DR). It is extremely important to recognize pre-proliferative retinopathy with its retinal signs, given that it may progress to proliferative retinopathy (new vessel formation).

Background retinopathy is the earliest stage of DR and is characterized by:

- capillary wall thickening;
- pericyte loss;
- increased leukocyte adhesion to the vessel wall;
- alteration in blood flow.

As the disease progresses, the retinal vessels become increasingly damaged, leading to progressive endothelial cell loss, which in turn results in the occlusion

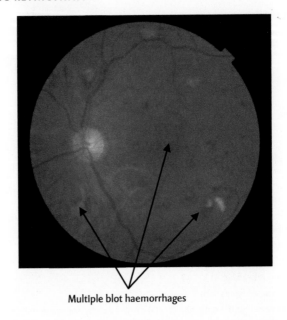

Multiple blot haemorrhages

Figure 7.1 A fundus photograph showing a retina with pre-proliferative retinopathy with multiple blot haemorrhages indicated.

(blockage) of retinal capillaries and the formation of extensive chronic retinal ischaemic areas. This is known as pre-proliferative retinopathy.

The current NHS Diabetic Eye Screening Programme (NHSDESP) grading criteria for R2 includes:

- Multiple blot haemorrhages (>8–10 per eye) (Figure 7.1).
- IRMA (Figure 7.2).
- Venous beading (Figure 7.3).
- Venous reduplication (Figure 7.4).

### 7.1.1 Multiple blot haemorrhages

These are large dark haemorrhages seen with a blot-like appearance, and are often referred to as strawberry- or raspberry-shaped haemorrhages. Noticeable differences between a dot and a blot are their size and irregular and indistinct borders. Provided the veins are not significantly dilated, the NHSDESP currently defines blot haemorrhages as haemorrhages larger than the width of the smallest of the four branches of the central retinal vein as they cross the edge of the disc, and consider pre-proliferative DR to be present when there are 8–10 blot

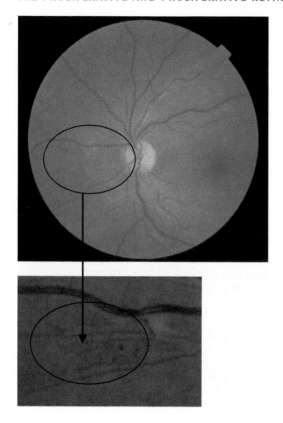

Figure 7.2 **Example of intra-retinal microvascular abnormalities (IRMA).**

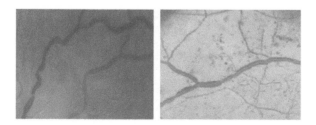

Figure 7.3 **Venous beading.**
Reproduced courtesy of Professor Paul M. Dodson and The Heart of England Retinal Screening Centre.

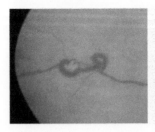 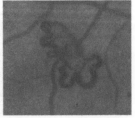

Figure 7.4 **Venous reduplication.**
Reproduced courtesy of Professor Paul M. Dodson and The Heart of England Retinal Screening Centre.

haemorrhages or more in total, across both macula and optic disc-centred retinal images of an eye. Blot haemorrhages are more sinister than dot haemorrhages as they occur in the deep layer of the retina and indicate retinal ischaemia; hence, it takes longer to resolve than superficial haemorrhage.

Flame haemorrhages are superficial haemorrhages in the nerve fibre layer. Flame-shaped haemorrhages should not be considered a feature of pre-proliferative retinopathy.

### 7.1.2 Intra-retinal microvascular abnormality

IRMA are believed to be either flat new vessels growing within the layer of the retina, rather than between the retina and the vitreous, or dilated remnants of capillaries within a large area of capillary occlusion. Where the capillary network becomes occluded, only remnants of perfused capillaries remain. IRMA become dilated (and visible) and tortuous in shape.

They can sometimes be mistaken for new vessels on the surface of the retina. The definitive test to differentiate between each type is by fluorescein angiography (a technique for examining the circulation of the retina using the dye tracing method) as IRMA do not leak.

IRMA are one of the defining features of severe non-proliferative DR based on the '4–2–1' criteria from the Early Treatment Diabetic Retinopathy Study (ETDRS). When comparing IRMA and NVE, IRMA are slightly larger in calibre and permeated in intra-retinal layers. In contrast, neovascularization or new vessels are finer, delicate, disorganized, and between the anterior surface of the retina and the posterior vitreous interface.

Other lesions, for example, collateral vessels caused by retinal vein occlusion can appear like IRMA. In cases where there is a well-localized patch of possible IRMA, the likelihood of collateral vessels due to retinal vein occlusion should be considered. If it is confirmed that small collateral vessels are present from a long-standing retinal vein occlusion, rather than IRMA, this should not be given an R2 grade.

### 7.1.3 Venous beading

Extensive capillary closure causes retina ischaemia resulting in the formation of venous beading and reduplication. These abnormalities always signify serious imminent risk of new vessel formation. They include venous beading and venous reduplication.

Venous beading (Figure 7.3) appears as irregular constriction and dilatation of the lumen (inner space of vessel) of retinal venules. It occurs due to hypoxia, which arises when there is extensive capillary occlusion and ischaemia. Initially, the veins may show focal areas of dilatation, but as the retinopathy progresses it may lead to significant venous beading.

Venous reduplication (Figure 7.4) is defined as dilatation of existing vessels adjacent to and approximately the same calibre as the originating vein. In appearance, they often look like a closed venous loop or a tangled knot. Again, they are associated with regions of retinal ischaemia.

## 7.2 NHSDESP guidelines for R2 referral

If the patient has features of pre-proliferative DR (R2), a routine referral should be made to the hospital eye service (HES) or digital surveillance to monitor the R2 changes. The ETDRS showed that very severe non-proliferative retinopathy (ETDRS 53E) had a 48.5% risk of progressing to high-risk proliferative diabetic retinopathy (PDR) within 1 year. It was recommended that even where follow-up was possible pan-retinal photocoagulation (PRP) treatment should be considered in these patients because they showed increased risk of severe visual loss (SVL) and the need for vitrectomy.

The NHSDESP standards for referral for pre-proliferative retinopathy are as follows:

> Achievable standard: 95% to be seen by an ophthalmologist within less than 13 weeks from the date of the screen (previously from referral outcome grader [ROG] date).

> Acceptable standard: 70% to be seen within 13 weeks from date of screening.

### 7.2.1 Pre-proliferative retinopathy and vision

Patients with pre-proliferative DR may not have visual symptoms; hence, the importance of screening to detect this stage of the disease. However, it has been reported that areas of significant retinal ischaemia correlate closely, although not always, to areas of reduced retinal sensitivity and, hence, visual field loss. The severity of the field loss has been shown to be variable, especially with age, with less severe visual field loss in younger patients.

However, in a recent survey of a cohort of patients with pre-proliferative DR in Birmingham, it was found that the majority of patients were referred in for ophthalmology assessment due to the coexistence of referable maculopathy over a 2-year follow-up period.

## 7.3 Proliferative retinopathy

The development of NVD and NVE on the retinal surface of the retina denotes the change from pre-proliferative retinopathy to the serious form proliferative retinopathy. New vessels arise from retinal ischaemia and are presumed to be an attempt of revascularization of hypoxic tissue. The short- and long-term consequences of new vessel formation are serious and affected patients may have a high risk of suffering severe visual loss. The significance of the new vessels is that they grow in the vitreo-retinal interface between the vitreous gel and retina, with no support from surrounding structures. As their vessel walls are fragile, they may fracture; hence, a rupture results in pre-retinal (in front of the retina) and vitreous haemorrhage. If advanced, new vessels may also grow on the iris, termed iris neovascularization.

### 7.3.1 Pathogenesis

The stimulus for pre-retinal new vessel growth is thought to be retinal hypoxia, caused by chronic retinal ischaemia, which in turn stimulates the release of VEGF. This protein is a primary mediator of retinal angiogenesis (the growth of new blood vessels from pre-existing vasculature).

VEGF was first discovered as a vascular permeability factor, but was subsequently recognized as an angiogenic factor and as a specific mitogen (a protein that triggers cells to undertake cell division) for vascular endothelial cells. Its mRNA and proteins are expressed in retinal cell types, including pericytes, astrocytes, glial cells, retinal pigment epithelial cells, and endothelial cells. It is released by these cells in response to hypoxia and binds with high-affinity VEGF receptors, expressed on vascular endothelial cells at the edge of the ischaemic area. This sets off a signalling cascade, which affects the survival, proliferation, and migration of endothelial cells, eventually leading to new vessel growth. In animal experiments, injection of VEGF into the vitreous can induce pre-retinal and iris neovascularization.

A study demonstrating VEGF levels using immunostaining techniques has shown that VEGF is absent or occurs in low levels in the majority of normal retinas. The VEGF level increases with pre-proliferative retinopathy, as the staining is of greater intensity, and it is shown to be highly elevated in diabetic patients with active proliferative retinopathy with intense staining in the retinal vessels, the choroid, and the ganglion cell layer.

It has been shown, however, that VEGF inhibition alone is insufficient to prevent retinal neovascularization. It has therefore been suggested that there are other mediators of retinal angiogenesis, such as growth hormone (GH), insulin-like growth factor-1 (IGF-1), angiotensins, erythropoietin, and fibroblast growth factor (FGF).

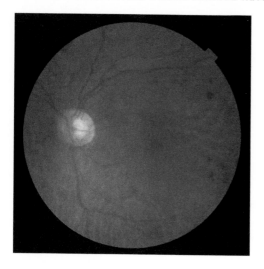

Figure 7.5 Example of NVD and NVE.

## 7.3.2 Retinal signs

The clinical signs of proliferative retinopathy are NVE or NVD, arising from the venous side of the circulation (Figure 7.5).

NVE occur away from the optic disc in the vascular arcades above and below the macula, and in the watershed areas temporal to the macula and in the nasal area. They invariably develop from the veins adjacent to areas of retinal ischaemia, arising in lacy networks of radiating spokes from vessels. They often cross over both the arteries and veins in the retina, indicating unregulated growth. Due to their fine calibre, they can be easily missed in retinal images. Untreated NVE, in particular, may be associated with retinal detachment, hence the importance of their early detection and treatment. If identified de novo, patients should have an urgent referral as they can either remain relatively stable, or grow rapidly and bleed.

A close-up view of NVE is given in Figure 7.6

NVD (Figure 7.7) or NVE should be referred urgently as they are at high risk of haemorrhage and, hence, threaten vision.

## 7.3.3 NHS Diabetic Eye Screening Programme guidelines

The classification consists of two categories—R3A (active proliferative retinopathy) and R3S (stable, treated proliferative retinopathy).

*Proliferative retinopathy (R3A)*

- NVE.
- Previous treatment has not been deemed stable by the treating ophthalmologist.

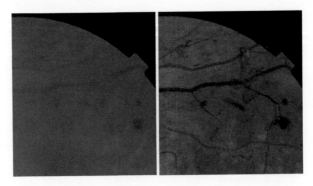

Figure 7.6 **New vessels elsewhere.**

- NVD.
- Pre-retinal/vitreous haemorrhage (see Chapter 8, 'Advanced diabetic eye disease').
- Patients where new features indicate reactivation of proliferation or potentially sight-threatening changes from fibrous proliferation, are seen with respect to a previously obtained reference image set.

If the patient has the features of R3A, an urgent referral to ophthalmology is required as there is a high risk of vitreous haemorrhage and development of advanced sight-threatening retinopathy.

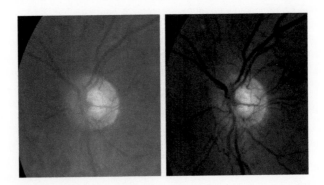

Figure 7.7 **New vessels at the optic disc.**
Reproduced courtesy of Professor Paul M. Dodson and The Heart of England Retinal Screening Centre.

*Proliferative retinopathy (R3S)*

- Evidence of peripheral retinal laser treatment and a stable retinal appearance with respect to reference images taken at or shortly after discharge from the HES.

A referral outcome grader (ROG) will always be responsible for the decision as to whether the presentation can be considered stable. A referral should be made as R3A in any case where there is doubt.

The NHSDESP standards for referral of new vessels state:

> Acceptable standard: 80% to be seen by an ophthalmologist within less than 6 weeks from the date of the retinal screening.

The severity of proliferative retinopathy can be classified by the presence or absence of high-risk characteristics for visual loss. The Diabetic Retinopathy Study (DRS) and ETDRS determined the high-risk characteristics. If an eye has three of the following four characteristics it is deemed as high risk:

- Presence of any neovascularization.
- Neovascularization on or within one disc diameter of the optic disc.
- A moderate to severe amount of neovascularization (greater than one-third of the disc area or NVE greater than half a disc area).
- Vitreous haemorrhage.

If untreated, 26% of patients with 'high risk' charcteristics and NVD will progress to severe visual loss within 2 years.

## 7.4 Summary

Pre-proliferative retinopathy heralds the development of more sinister proliferative changes, which may threaten vision. Referral should be made so these patients can be closely monitored. The new finding of proliferative retinopathy in a diabetic patient is an urgent referral to eye services as pre-retinal and vitreous haemorrhage may be imminent; the latter may obscure the retinal view for many months, preventing laser treatment. Before the digital camera screening programme, a UK national audit of referrals to diabetic eye clinics indicated that 25% of patients with proliferative retinopathy were presenting at a late stage with visual symptoms (due to vitreous haemorrhage). This reinforces the importance of accurate retinal screening.

FURTHER READING

Anon. (1978). Photocoagulation treatment of proliferative diabetic retinopathy: the second report of diabetic retinopathy study findings. *Ophthalmology* **85**: 82–106.

Bek T. (1999) Venous loops and reduplications in diabetic retinopathy. Prevalence, distribution, and pattern of development. *Acta Ophthalmol Scand* **77**: 130–4.

Boulton M, Foreman D, Williams G, McLeod D. (1998). VEGF localisation in diabetic retinopathy. *Br J Ophthalmol* **82**: 561–8.

Chee CKL, Flanagan DW. (1993). Visual field loss with capillary non-perfusion in preproliferative and early proliferative diabetic retinopathy. *Br J Ophthalmol* **77**: 726–30.

Davis MD, Fisher MR, Gangnon RE, Barton F, Aiello LM, Chew EY, et al. (1998). Risk factors for high-risk proliferative diabetic retinopathy and severe visual loss: Early Treatment Diabetic Retinopathy Study report number 18. *Invest Ophthalmol Vis Sci* **39**: 233–52.

Diabetic Retinopathy Study Research Group. (1981). Photocoagulation treatment of proliferative diabetic retinopathy: Clinical application of Diabetic Retinopathy Study (DRS) findings: DRS Report Number 8. *Ophthalmology* **88**: 583–600.

Gangnon RE, Davis MD, Hubbard LD, Aiello LM, Chew EY, Ferris FL 3rd, et al. (2008). Early Treatment Diabetic Retinopathy Study Research Group. A severity scale for diabetic macular edema developed from ETDRS data. *Invest Ophthalmol Vis Sci* **49**(11): 5041–7.

Kohner EM. (1993). Diabetic retinopathy. *Br Med J* **307**: 1195–9.

Livingstone C, Ferns G. (2003). Insulin-like growth factor-related proteins and diabetic complications. *Br J Diabetes Vasc Dis* **3**(5): 326–9.

Mitamura Y, Harada C, Harada T. (2005). Role of cytokines and trophic factors in the pathogenesis of diabetic retinopathy. *Curr Diabetes Rev* **1**: 73–81. http://citeseerx.ist.psu.edu/viewdoc/download?doi=10.1.1.324.7536&rep=rep1&type=pdf (accessed 18 August 2019).

Schultz GS, Grant MB. (1991). Neovascular growth factors. *Eye* **5**: 170–80.

Shin YW, Lee YJ, Lee BR, Cho HY. (2009). Effects of an intravitreal bevacizumab injection combined with panretinal photocoagulation on high-risk proliferative diabetic retinopathy. *Korean J Ophthalmol* **23**(4): 266–72.

Watanabe D, Suzuma K, Matsui S, Kurimoto M, Kiryu J, Kita M, et al. (2005). Erythropoietin as a retinal angiogenic factor in proliferative diabetic retinopathy. *N Engl J Med* **353**: 782–92.

# Advanced diabetic eye disease

Karen Whitehouse

---

**KEY POINTS**

- Advanced diabetic eye disease can remain asymptomatic for a long time, due to the slow progression of proliferative retinopathy, and the fact that the macula may not be affected.
- Diabetic retinopathy screening is an important factor in intervention and treatment.
- The grading criteria for advanced disease (R3) as defined by the NHS Diabetic Eye Screening Programme (NHSDESP) is discussed, as well as the management of the patient and subsequent treatment regimen.
- This chapter examines the progression of proliferative disease and its' natural history if left untreated.

---

## 8.1 Introduction

Advanced diabetic eye disease may be classed as end-stage damage from diabetic retinopathy. Both Type 1 and Type 2 patients are at risk.

Microvascular complications of diabetes include increased vascular permeability, ischaemia, and formation of new vessels (neovascularization). Neovascularization of the retina generates a high risk of vitreous haemorrhage and fibrosis; the leading causes of persistent severe visual loss is vitreous or pre-retinal haemorrhage, macular oedema/pigmentary changes associated with macular oedema, and retinal detachment. The incidence of severe visual loss can be reduced with laser photocoagulation and vitrectomy surgery.

The NHSDESP protocol states that retinopathy screeners/graders should not enter into detailed dialogue with the patient about the results of their screening, as a qualified grader should assess and confirm advanced disease. However, it is appropriate that, if a patient needs urgent referral, they will need to be advised of this as soon as it is known in order to ensure that they can make themselves available at short notice for treatment. The screener should ensure that the patient's contact details are accurate should they need to be contacted quickly. Programmes will have local protocol for screeners to follow.

## 8.2 Subhyaloid/pre-retinal haemorrhages

Vascular endothelial growth factor (VEGF) is an endothelial cell-specific angiogenic factor and plays a major part in intra-ocular neovascularization. As VEGF production is also stimulated by high glucose levels, it is therefore as likely that patients with Type 1 and Type 2 diabetes are susceptible long-term. Most new vessels arise from veins in a characteristic pattern, forming loops or a fine irregular meshwork—sometimes referred to as 'butterfly wing'. In eyes with widespread ischaemia, new vessels at the optic disc (NVD) may arise.

The vitreous humour is an inert, transparent gel, filling the majority of the posterior segment of the eye. New vessels grow forward from the retina, bridging towards the posterior surface of the vitreous; the vessels are fragile and disrupted easily by traction within the vitreous, which will cause the fragile vessels to bleed.

As haemorrhage forms, they take on a characteristic appearance with a fluid level (Figure 8.1) due to gravity. The patient may complain of floaters or 'spots' in the vision. The condition is not due to bleeding of the vitreous humour, but rather bleeding from the retinal vessels.

The screener/grader may be presented with a haemorrhage with a horizontal gravitational level at the superior surface, which obscures the underlying retina, as red cells settle within the cavity of the haemorrhage. The profile may be disturbed depending upon the posture of the patient. The screener/grader will grade this as R3A (as in proliferative retinopathy), as new vessels may be masked by the pre-retinal haemorrhage, and therefore a recommendation for urgent referral should be made to the hospital eye service (HES), as per NHSDESP standards .

The haemorrhage may occur either in the level of the subhyaloid space between the posterior vitreous face and retina (pre-retinal haemorrhage, see Figure 8.1), or under the internal limiting membrane resulting in a subhyaloid haemorrhage.

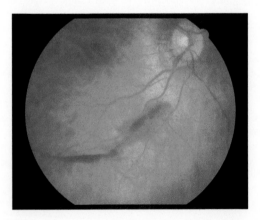

Figure 8.1 Pre-retinal haemorrhage, which is developing a typical gravitational level.

If the pre-retinal haemorrhage is large it can break through into the vitreous humour, causing a vitreous haemorrhage.

## 8.3 Vitreous haemorrhage

Between 31 and 54% of vitreous haemorrhages are due to diabetic retinopathy (DR). Sight-threatening vitreous haemorrhage occurs abruptly and painlessly. In the early stages, the patient may complain of a sudden onset of floaters, or a cobweb image across their vision, or the vision may become reddened and hazy. However,

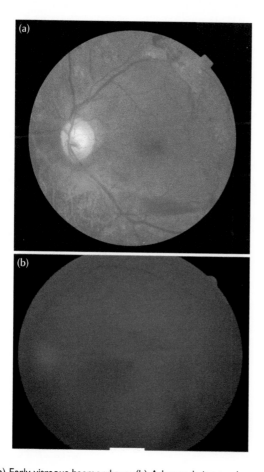

Figure 8.2 (a) Early vitreous haemorrhage. (b) Advanced vitreous haemorrhage.

(b) Reproduced courtesy of Professor Paul M. Dodson and The Heart of England Retinal Screening Centre.

severe or advanced haemorrhage can compromise visual acuity dramatically causing areas of diminished sight within the visual field (scotomas) or profound visual loss. The patient may note that the vision is worse when lying in a prone position, due to haemorrhage shifting within the vitreous and obscuring the macula.

The screener/grader will be presented with a red haze obscuring the retinal blood vessels and/or the optic nerve, indicating a less severe haemorrhage (Figure 8.2(a)), or a dense red fundus with an indistinct detail of retinal blood vessels and the optic nerve, which indicates a severe vitreous haemorrhage (Figure 8.2(b)). All cases of vitreous haemorrhage will be graded as R3A—an urgent referral.

Vitreous haemorrhage slowly resolves at a rate of approximately 1% per day, clearing more quickly in vitrectomized eyes and more slowly in younger eyes, but it does take many months to resolve. However, the underlying proliferative retinopathy may cause further repeated haemorrhages, such that vision does not improve and retinal examination is not possible. This is one of the major indications for vitrectomy surgery.

## 8.4 Gliosis

As the disease develops further, the process of neovascularization causes scarring (gliosis), as fibrous tissue develops around the new vessels. The fibrous tissue may eventually contract and develop into tractional retinal detachment. The screener/grader will be presented with fibrous strands emanating from the new vessel glial complex, which once large is immobile (Figure 8.3). The NHS screening programme grade for this appearance is still R3A with an urgent referral outcome.

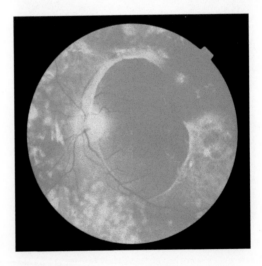

Figure 8.3 Gliosis with pan-retinal photocoagulation.

CHAPTER 8

## 8.5 Tractional retinal detachment

Proliferative diabetic retinopathy is the primary causative factor in tractional retinal detachments. Detachments are a major complication, due to the new vessels contracting, and subsequently pulling the retina from the underlying retinal pigment epithelium (RPE); the resulting fibrosis will primarily consist of RPE cells. Studies suggest that soluble vascular cell adhesion molecules may contribute to progression of neovascularization and fibrosis, as a result of endothelial and retinal pigment epithelial cell activation. Retinal detachment also augments the existing inflammation within the diabetic retina.

Tractional retinal detachments develop slowly, progressing as fibrovascular proliferation increases. Peripheral tractional detachments are therefore rarely, if ever, noticed by the patient. Macular tractional detachments, on the other hand, tend to be symptomatic, as visual acuity will be affected. The patient may complain of a veiled effect or 'curtain' across their field of vision; if the macula is affected, they may notice that straight lines appear distorted. The highest elevation of the retina occurs at the traction site and vessels are pulled towards the adhesions.

The screener will therefore be presented with a retinal view of concave fibrovascular bands and smooth-surfaced detachments. Tractional detachments are opaque and immobile (Figure 8.4).

The NHS diabetic retinopathy grade is R3A with an urgent referral necessary. If the patient presents with sudden loss of vision, they will be referred to an ophthalmologist the same day, as an emergency.

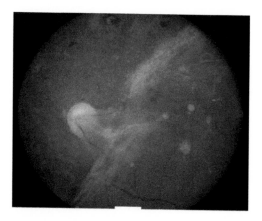

Figure 8.4 Tractional retinal detachment at the optic disc.
Reproduced courtesy of Professor Paul M. Dodson and The Heart of England Retinal Screening Centre.

## 8.6 Neovascular glaucoma due to iris new vessels

In cases of advanced proliferative retinopathy, vascular proliferation may extend into the anterior chamber on the surface of the iris (iris new vessels, see Section 8.7, 'Rubeosis Iridis'). This results in new vessels and accompanying fibrous membrane growing, causing obstruction to fluid drainage by blocking the canal of Schlemm and, hence, raising intra-ocular pressure. This, in turn, causes the cornea to become oedematous, and the optic nerve, affected by the high intra-ocular pressure, becomes atrophic. If the disease develops, the fibrous membrane contracts causing synaechiae—adhesion of the iris to the cornea or of the iris to the lens.

The patient will present with a red, acutely painful eye, due to the high intra-ocular pressure, and often there is significant loss of vision. The screener must undertake an anterior chamber view to show visible neovascularization of the iris. The condition will subsequently be diagnosed via slit lamp examination and intra-ocular pressure measurement. This is an ocular emergency to obtain analgesia and treatment to lower the high intra-ocular pressure. (The formal grading level remains as R3A.) This condition is fortunately rarely identified in the national diabetic retinopathy screening programme.

## 8.7 Rubeosis Iridis

In cases of severe proliferative retinopathy, vascular proliferation extends into the posterior iris, through the pupil, along the anterior surface of the iris, and then into the angle. The resulting new vessels in the iris are termed iris neovascularization or iris rubeosis.

The screener should take an anterior chamber view of an undilated pupil in order to demonstrate iris new vessels; these may be evident or may show as diffuse reddening of the iris. They may be visible as small groups of blood vessels along the pupillary margin or in the anterior chamber angle (Figure 8.5).

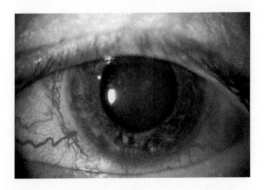

Figure 8.5 Rubeosis Iridis with corneal haze.

The grader will class the grade as R3A and urgently refer the patient on the same day to ophthalmology services if the condition has not previously been diagnosed and treated.

## 8.8 Summary

In synopsis, the current NHSDESP benchmark standards state that the acceptable threshold level for people referred to the HES with a final grading outcome of R3A in the worst eye, attending a first consultation in the HES within 6 weeks of their screening or surveillance event, is ≥80.0%. The HES appointment can occur outside the reporting period, but must occur within 6 weeks of the screening or surveillance event.

### 8.8.1 Performance thresholds

Patients presenting with sudden loss of vision should be referred immediately to their local Eye Accident and Emergency or, if possible, to the HES.

FURTHER READING

Berdahl JP, Mruthyunjaya PMD; Ed. by Scott IU, Fekrat S. (2007). *Vitreous hemorrhage: diagnosis and treatment*. American Academy Ophthalmology

Fong DS, Ferris FL 3rd, Davis MD, Chew EY. (1999). Causes of severe visual loss in the early treatment diabetic retinopathy study: ETDRS report no. 24. *Am J Ophthalmol* **127**(2): 137–41.

Nork TM, Wallow IH, Sramek SJ, Anderson G. (1987). Müller's cell involvement in proliferative diabetic retinopathy. *Arch Ophthalmol* **105**(10): 1424–9.

Ray D, Mishra M, Ralph S, Read I, Davies R, Brenchley P. (2004). Association of the VEGF gene with proliferative diabetic retinopathy but not proteinuria in diabetes. *Diabetes* **53**(3): 861–4. American Diabetes Association. https://diabetes.diabetesjournals.org/content/53/3/861 (accessed 20 August 2019).

Limb GA, Hickman-Casey J, Hollifield RD, Chignell AH. (1999). Vascular adhesion molecules in vitreous from eyes with proliferative diabetic retinopathy. *Chignell Investig Ophthalmol Visual Sci* **40**: 2453–7.

Negi A, Vernon SA. (2003). An overview of the eye in diabetes. *J Roy Soc Med* **96**: 266–72.

Gov.UK. (2012). Diabetic eye screening: retinal image grading criteria. https://www.gov.uk/government/publications/diabetic-eye-screening-retinal-image-grading-criteria (accessed 18 August 2019).

Gov.UK. (2018). Diabetic eye screening key performance indicators for 2018 to 2019: definitions. https://www.gov.uk/government/publications/nhs-population-screening-reporting-data-definitions/diabetic-eye-screening-key-performance-indicators-for-2018-to-2019-definitions (accessed 18 August 2019).

Gov.UK. (2019). Diabetic eye screening programme: pathway standards. https://www.gov.uk/government/publications/diabetic-eye-screening-programme-standards (accessed 20 August 2019).

# Other ophthalmic lesions in the fundus

Jonathan M. Gibson

**KEY POINTS**

- Diabetic retinopathy (DR) screening will detect other ophthalmic conditions, some of which may be important.
- Pattern recognition by the grader and local management protocols are very helpful.
- Retinal vascular disorders, retinal drusen, choroidal naevi, asteroid hyalosis, and age-related macular degeneration (AMD) are commonly detected.

## 9.1 Introduction

Retinal screening of patients with digital fundus photography throws up a number of images that are puzzling for the grader, and these may represent harmless variations of normality or serious ophthalmic pathology. In this chapter, examples of the common and important abnormalities that might be detected and details on what to do about them are given.

## 9.2 Retinal drusen and age-related macular degeneration (AMD)

Retinal drusen are a common finding in elderly patients and represent age-related changes in Bruch's membrane, the basement membrane of the retinal pigment epithelium. They are, therefore, situated under the retina and appear as discrete yellowish lesions (see Figures 9.1 and 9.2).

The importance of drusen in the context of DR lies in differentiating them from diabetic retinal exudates. They are a manifestation of dry AMD and the soft types can predispose to the formation of choroidal neovascular membrane and the loss of central vision (Table 9.1).

Wet AMD is the commonest cause of visual loss in the population over the age of 60 and the commonest cause of blindness in diabetic subjects in the UK. The dry type is more common with several phenotypical variants, such as pigmentary

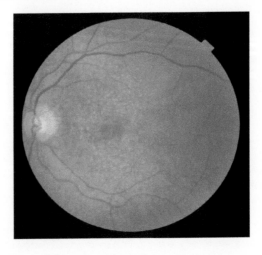

Figure 9.1 Retinal drusen in typical appearance.

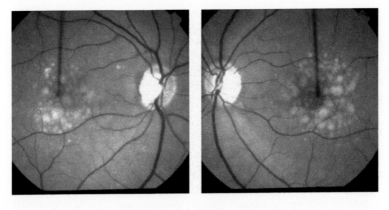

Figure 9.2 Red-free fundus photographs of right and left eyes in the same patient showing soft retinal drusen at the macula and the symmetrical position in each eye.

changes, atrophy, and thinning, leading on to geographic atrophy. Wet macular degeneration can cause significant visual loss over a short period (Figure 9.3). This is due to the growth of new vessels and due to vascular endothelial growth factor (VEGF), beneath the retinal pigment epithelium (RPE; see Figure 9.4), and therefore signs of haemorrhage and oedema are sub-retinal. The early signs can

**Table 9.1** Comparison of main features of retinal drusen and exudates

| Criteria | Drusen | Exudates |
|---|---|---|
| Colour | Yellow | Creamy white |
| Edges | Tend to be soft | Tend to be hard |
| Symmetry between eyes | Always symmetrical | Occasionally symmetrical |
| Situation in fundus | Always at macula | Can be anywhere—often circinate |
| Which layer of retina | Sub-retinal in the RPE (Figure 9.4) | Intra-retinal (Figure 9.4) |

be subtle, with just an abnormal appearance to the foveal area. If wet AMD is detected by screening, it is usually accompanied by changes in central vision, and warrants an early or urgent referral. (In the UK there is a fast-track referral pathway with subjects being seen within 2 weeks.)

Patients in whom retinal drusen are detected on screening do not require referral to the eye clinic, unless the patient is known to be suffering from visual symptoms, of which distortion of images is the most important.

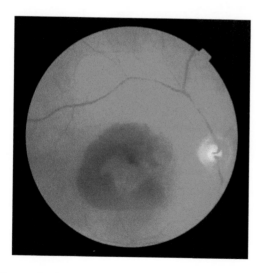

Figure 9.3 Wet macular degeneration: large macular haemorrhage (note sub-retinal) with a grey area showing the choroidal neovascular membrane.

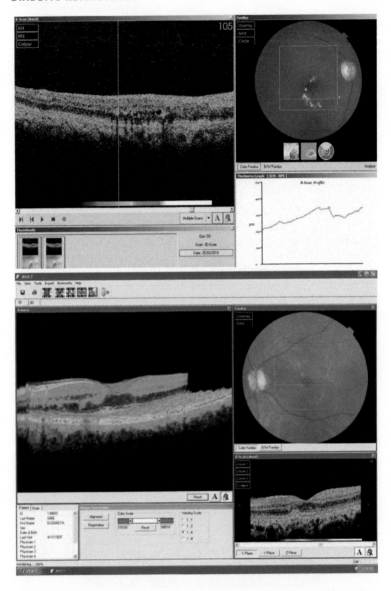

Figure 9.4 Upper panel shows the optical coherence tomography appearance of exudates occurring in the mid layers of the retina. Lower panel shows typical appearance of drusen occurring in and arising from the RPE.

CHAPTER 9

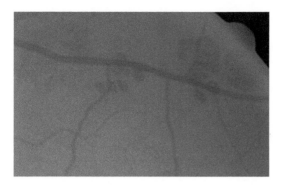

Figure 9.5 **Bear-track pigmentation in the superotemporal quadrant.**
Reproduced courtesy of Professor Paul M. Dodson and The Heart of England Retinal Screening Centre.

## 9.3 Abnormalities of fundus pigmentation

### 9.3.1 Congenital pigmentation of the retina

This may occur as congenital hypertrophy of the retinal pigment epithelium (CHRPE) or as a characteristic bear-track pigmentation, which looks like a trail of muddy footprints (Figure 9.5). These are both harmless findings, although CHRPE, when in large numbers or bilateral, have been associated with familial polyposis coli in susceptible individuals.

### 9.3.2 Acquired pigmented lesions

This may occur from choroidal naevi and tumours, previous inflammatory disease of the choroid and retina, and from pre-existing laser scars (Figure 9.6).

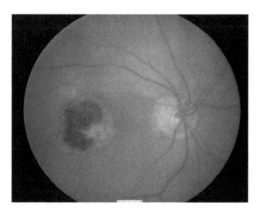

Figure 9.6 **Pigmentation from heavy macular laser photocoagulation 10 years earlier.**
Reproduced courtesy of Professor Paul M. Dodson and The Heart of England Retinal Screening Centre.

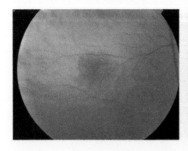 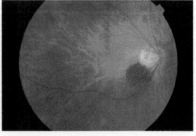

Figure 9.7 Choroidal naevi in separate patients. The lesion adjacent to the disc is suspicious and should be referred to the ophthalmology clinic.
Reproduced courtesy of Professor Paul M. Dodson and The Heart of England Retinal Screening Centre.

Choroidal naevi are a common finding in Caucasians and are estimated to occur in up to 5% of the population. They are benign melanocytic tumours, but rarely may become malignant, and it is estimated that the annual rate of malignant transformation is about 1 in 8800 cases. The main significance of choroidal naevi is to distinguish them from malignant melanoma of the choroid (Figure 9.7). Signs of malignant change in naevi may be subtle, but the following mnemonic can be helpful and has been formulated by ocular oncology experts in the USA.

## 9.4 'To find small ocular melanoma using helpful hints daily'

In the absence of any of the features in Table 9.2, the lesion is unlikely to be a malignant melanoma. However, it may be difficult for the grader or screener to appreciate all the above features from two-dimensional retinal photographs alone and, in general, it is advisable to gain advice on the policy of referral of suspicious lesions from the local ophthalmologists.

Management of choroidal naevi that are not suspicious is usually by means of serial fundus photography by the local referring optometrist or by the hospital eye department.

| Table 9.2 | 'To find small ocular melanoma using helpful hints daily' | |
|---|---|---|
| • T | To | Thickness (>2 mm) |
| • F | Find | Fluid (sub-retinal) |
| • S | Small | Symptoms |
| • O | Ocular | Orange pigment (lipofuscin in the lesion) |
| • M | Melanoma | Margin less than 3 mm from optic disc |
| • UH | Using helpful | Ultrasonography hollowness |
| • H | Hints | Halo absence |
| • D | Daily | Drusen absence |

Source: Adapted with permission from Kaliki S and Shields C.L. Uveal melanoma: relatively rare but deadly cancer. *Eye*, **31** (2): 241–257. Copyright © 2016, Springer Nature. Source data from: Shields CL, Furuta M, Berman EL, Zahler JD, Hoberman DM, Dinh DH et al. Choroidal nevus transformation into melanoma: analysis of 2514 consecutive cases. *Arch Ophthalmol* 2009; 127(8): 981–987; Collaborative Ocular Melanoma Study Group. Factors predictive of growth and treatment of small choroidal melanoma: COMS Report No. 5. *Arch Ophthalmol* 1997; 115: 1537–1544.

### 9.4.1 Myelinated nerve fibres

These occur when the normal process of myelination of the optic nerve continues beyond the lamina cribrosa into the retinal nerve fibres. They have a characteristic creamy white appearance (Figure 9.8), with a feathery margin at the peripheral part of the lesion and are generally a harmless finding, requiring no further investigation.

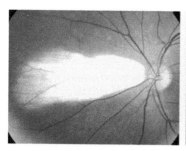 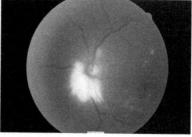

Figure 9.8 **Myelinated nerve fibres.**
Reproduced courtesy of Professor Paul M. Dodson and The Heart of England Retinal Screening Centre.

### 9.4.2 Myopia

There are a number of fundal appearances associated with myopia, which are harmless. These range from pale areas of choroido-retinal atrophy around the optic disc, the so-called myopic crescent, to areas of pale streaks corresponding to ruptures in Bruch's membrane, the basement membrane of the retina. These latter abnormalities are termed 'lacquer cracks' (Figure 9.9).

Occasionally, the defects caused by the myopia can cause growth of sub-retinal blood vessels, representing a choroidal neovascular membrane and, therefore, any associated macular haemorrhage in myopic fundi should be treated with suspicion and referred to the ophthalmologists for tertiary grading or to the eye clinic.

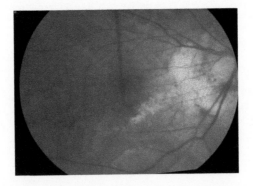

Figure 9.9 Fundus of a highly myopic patient showing peri-papillary atrophic and pigmentary changes, and a single lacquer crack extending inferior to the macula.
Reproduced courtesy of Professor Paul M. Dodson and The Heart of England Retinal Screening Centre.

### 9.4.3 Laser photocoagulation scars

Laser photocoagulation reactions are seen immediately as greyish-white discrete lesions, but within a few weeks pigmentary and atrophic changes start to become visible. Reactions may be predominantly atrophic or pigmented (see Figures 9.6 and 9.10).

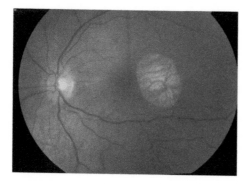

Figure 9.10 Laser photocoagulation scar from previous treatment for wet macular degeneration 5 years earlier. Atrophy of the retinal pigment epithelium shows visible underlying large choroidal blood vessels and sclera.
Reproduced courtesy of Professor Paul M. Dodson and The Heart of England Retinal Screening Centre.

## 9.5 Inflammatory disease

Previous inactive choroiditis and retinitis scars are commonly seen in fundus photographs, but it may be impossible to determine a cause and, in many cases, they represent long-standing childhood or congenital lesions. Active inflammatory lesions are most unlikely to be detected by retinal screening for DR because patients would notice reduced vision and other symptoms. Signs of active inflammation are very hazy pictures, as a result of associated vitritis, and haemorrhage and

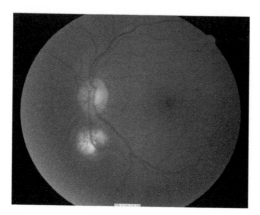

Figure 9.11 Single scar presumed to be due to congenital toxoplasmosis.
Reproduced courtesy of Professor Paul M. Dodson and The Heart of England Retinal Screening Centre.

fuzzy white, creamy lesions in the fundus. Suspected cases should be referred to the ophthalmologist for urgent investigation.

Toxoplasmosis is probably the most common infectious disease involving the retina and is caused by *Toxoplasma gondii*, a sporozoan parasite with a two-host life cycle. Congenital infection or acquired infection in immunocompromised individuals can be associated with retinal infection (a retinitis). Inactive healed lesions are the ones most likely to be found in retinopathy screening and the characteristic appearance is of a large, well-defined scar surrounded by pigment (Figures 9.11 and 9.12).

Common causes of inflammatory scars due to retinitis are toxoplasmosis, toxocariasis, syphilis, and herpes virus infections, including cytomegalovirus. An important cause of choroidal infection is tuberculosis.

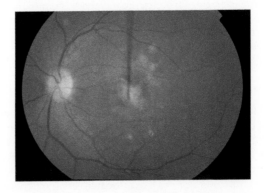

Figure 9.12 Fundus showing multifocal scars and subretinal fibrosis under the fovea. This is a case of inactive multifocal choroiditis.

Reproduced courtesy of Professor Paul M. Dodson and The Heart of England Retinal Screening Centre.

## 9.6 Retinovascular disorders

The commonest retinovascular disorders that are likely to be detected during screening photography are branch and central retinal vein occlusions, and retinal artery macroaneurysms.

### 9.6.1 Branch retinal vein occlusion

Branch retinal vein occlusion (BRVO) occurs at crossing points, where a retinal vein and arteriole share a common adventitial sheath. In most cases, the arteriole is anterior to the corresponding vein and compression of the vein causes an occlusion. Cases are classified depending on the size of the vein occluded and

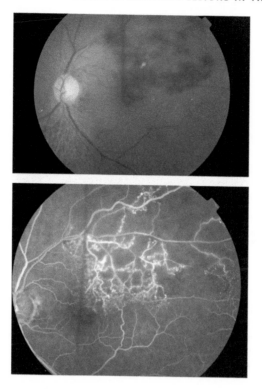

Figure 9.13 Superotemporal branch retinal vein occlusion on fundus photography and fluorescein angiogram, showing retinal haemorrhages and single cotton wool spot in the acute phase, and associated capillary fall-out on angiography. Vision was 6/9.
Reproduced courtesy of Professor Paul M. Dodson and The Heart of England Retinal Screening Centre.

can vary from a small occlusion affecting the macula to a whole quadrant of the fundus, the superotemporal being the most likely to be affected (Figure 9.13). If the macula is involved, vision is invariably affected, but the prognosis in the longer term depends on how much associated ischaemic damage occurs to the capillary circulation at the macula.

Clinical features are variable and patients may be asymptomatic if the macula is not involved. Haemorrhages are flame-shaped, dot and blot, and in more severe cases, confluent and of a dark colour. Other findings are cotton wool spots, dilated retinal veins in the affected quadrant, exudates (chronic phase), and pigment

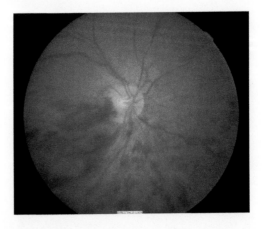

Figure 9.14 Inferior, hemi-central retinal vein occlusion with haemorrhages and multiple cotton wool spots visible.

disturbance, and collateral vessels may occur. Fluorescein angiography (FFA) may be useful in assessing which cases may require laser treatment.

Management of BRVO consists of investigation as to the cause and modification of any underlying medical risk factors, of which systemic hypertension is most common. Ophthalmic treatment is indicated if there is macular oedema, visual acuity (VA) of 6/12 or worse, and no spontaneous improvement in 3–6 months. Macular grid laser treatment and intra-vitreal injections of anti-VEGF agents are the mainstay of treatment for macular oedema, and sectoral pan-retinal photocoagulation laser treatment may be required for retinal neovascularization. About 50% of cases will spontaneously settle and achieve vision of 6/12 or better.

### 9.6.2 Central retinal vein occlusion

Central retinal vein occlusion (CRVO) and hemi-CRVO (see Figures 9.14 and 9.15) occur when the central retinal vein is occluded posterior to the cribriform plate. They are classified clinically as ischaemic and non-ischaemic on the basis of fundus examination and fluorescein angiographic findings.

All patients with BRVO and CRVO require investigation, which should include blood pressure (BP), full blood count (FBC), erythrocyte sedimentation ratio (ESR), urea and electrolytes (U&E), glucose, lipids, protein electrophoresis, thyroid function tests (TFTs), and electrocardiogram (ECG). Patients should be referred for an ophthalmologist's opinion as soon as possible for investigation and possible treatment. Management of CRVO will depend on whether it is classified as ischaemic or non-ischaemic; this is based on clinical examination and, in some cases, fluorescein angiography.

It is important to treat any underlying medical conditions to prevent recurrence in the fellow eye; this is best achieved by the ophthalmologist liaising with

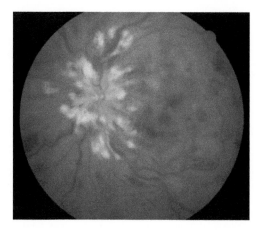

Figure 9.15 Ischaemic CRVO with haemorrhages in all four quadrants, cotton wool spots, and dilated veins.

a physician. Treatment options include management of raised intra-ocular pressure, laser pan-retinal photocoagulation (PRP), and intra-vitreal injection of anti-VEGF agents.

### 9.6.3 Retinal arterial occlusion

These are ophthalmic emergencies, which present with sudden loss of vision (see Chapter 4, 'Diabetes and the eye', and Figure 4.3). They are most unlikely to present to the screening programme because of this and they require urgent medical care.

### 9.6.4 Retinal arteriolar emboli

Emboli in the retinal arterioles are a common finding in fundus photographs and the majority are asymptomatic (see Figure 9.16). Prevalence rates of 1.3% have been reported in older white populations, but it is probably lower in non-white populations. They may originate from the carotid arteries associated with atherosclerosis or, more rarely, they may originate from the heart. The commonest appearance, the cholesterol embolus or Hollenhorst plaque, is of a highly refractile lesion within an arteriole, commonly at a bifurcation in the vessel.

A yellow refractile lesion is usually seen at the arteriolar bifurcation embolus, but in the case shown in Figure 9.16 has travelled further along the retinal arteriole.

Patients in whom an embolus is detected should be referred to a physician for further medical investigation as the patient is at risk of myocardial infarction, cerebrovascular emboli and stroke, or renal damage. Diagnosis is made by the

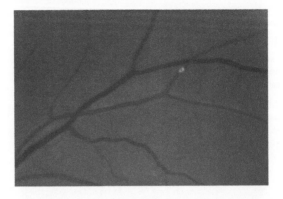

Figure 9.16 A yellow refractile lesion is usually seen at the arteriolar bifurcation embolus, but in this case it has travelled further along the retinal arteriole.
Reproduced courtesy of Professor Paul M. Dodson and The Heart of England Retinal Screening Centre.

history and special investigations, including Doppler scanning of the carotid arteries. Management involves reducing the risk of emboli being shed with medication and/or surgery to the carotid arteries.

### 9.6.5 Hypertensive retinopathy

Systemic hypertension is one of the commonest diseases of the Western world and is commonly found in patients with diabetes mellitus. Ophthalmic features are focal narrowing and irregularity of the retinal arterioles, and in more severe cases cotton wool spots and retinal haemorrhages, both flame-shaped in

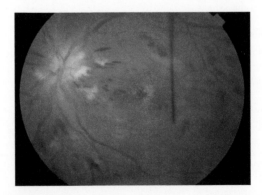

Figure 9.17 Accelerated hypertension in a patient sent for DR screening and with BP of 230/140 mmHg.
Reproduced courtesy of Professor Paul M. Dodson and The Heart of England Retinal Screening Centre.

**Table 9.3** Grading for hypertensive retinopathy

| Grade | Retinal changes | Hypertension severity | Prognosis |
|-------|-----------------|----------------------|-----------|
| A | Arteriolar narrowing, focal constriction | Non-malignant | Depends on BP, age, other risk factors, and end-organ damage |
| B | Haemorrhages, exudates cotton wool spots +/− papilloedema | Accelerated/ malignant | 80% dead in 2 years if not treated. Prognosis depends on BP control |

the nerve-fibre layer and deeper blot haemorrhages (Figure 9.17). It should be noted that arteriovenous nipping or nicking is more usually considered to be a sign of arteriosclerotic disease, although this commonly coexists with hypertensive changes.

Accelerated hypertension (Figure 9.17) occurs when the BP is severely raised, for example >220 mmHg systolic and >120 mmHg diastolic pressures. Fundal features are as described before, but with optic disc swelling and exudates in a star pattern at the macula. Patients in this category should be referred urgently.

The original classification of hypertensive retinopathy by Keith, Wagener, and Barker in 1939 was based on correlation of the fundus findings, and the severity of hypertension and survival risk of the patient. More recent grading schemes have tried to recognize the modern change in survival rates of patients and have reflected this in simplified schemes (see Table 9.3).

### 9.6.6 Macroaneurysms

Retinal arteriolar macroaneurysms are focal dilatations of retinal arterioles and are much larger than microaneurysms, usually 100–250 µm in size. They are often asymptomatic, but vision can be threatened by slow exudative decompensation of the lesion, which can threaten the macula, or from acute haemorrhage (Figure 9.18). Haemorrhage from macroaneurysms is unusual in that it can occur in sub-retinal, intra-retinal, and pre-retinal planes, as well as breaking through into the vitreous.

Macroaneurysms are associated most commonly with systemic hypertension, but may also be associated with carotid artery disease, and patients in whom asymptomatic lesions are found should be referred to a physician for further investigation.

In most cases, spontaneous resolution occurs, but if the vision is threatened retinal focal laser photocoagulation either directly to seal off the macroaneurysm or indirectly around the lesion can be performed. Anti-VEGF injections have also been tried successfully when associated with exudation.

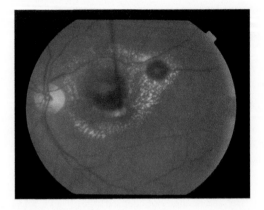

Figure 9.18 Two retinal arteriolar macroaneurysms arising from the same retinal vessel.
Reproduced courtesy of Professor Paul M. Dodson and The Heart of England Retinal Screening Centre.

## 9.7 Rarer abnormalities

Anomalous vascular patterns in the retina may occur with vessels encroaching and crossing the macular region and crossing the horizontal raphe (the imaginary continued line from the optic disc to the fovea). These abnormal vascular patterns are usually congenital and asymptomatic, although the abnormal vessels are more likely to develop pathological changes, presumably due to abnormal blood flow.

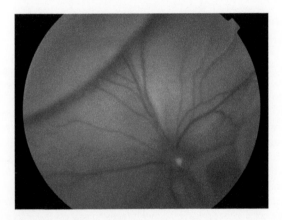

Figure 9.19 Bullous retinal detachment with a large area of serous retinal detachment.
Reproduced courtesy of Professor Paul M. Dodson and The Heart of England Retinal Screening Centre.

## 9.7.1 Retinal detachment

These are usually symptomatic and would usually present as an emergency to the ophthalmic department with loss of vision. If the macula is attached, however, central vision will be unaffected and the patient may be unaware (Figure 9.19).

## 9.7.2 Asteroid hyalosis

This common condition, which is caused by degenerative changes in the vitreous gel, gives the appearance of multiple reflective floaters in front of the retina and may move on sequential photography. If the condition is marked as in the example given here, fundus photography may not be able to show the retina clearly. In most cases, this is a harmless asymptomatic condition, but if fundus photography is poor, the patient should be referred to the eye clinic for examination (Figure 9.20).

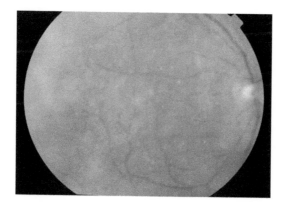

Figure 9.20  A case of asteroides hyalosis with poor retinal visualization that required referral to the eye clinic for annual DR screening.

Reproduced courtesy of Professor Paul M. Dodson and The Heart of England Retinal Screening Centre.

FURTHER READING

Kaliki S, Shields CL. (2017). Uveal melanoma: relatively rare but deadly cancer. *Eye (Lond)* 31(2): 241–57.

Denniston AKO, Murray PI. (2018). *Oxford Handbook of Ophthalmology*. Oxford University Press, Oxford.

Freund KB, Sarraf D, Mieler W, Yannuzzi L. (2016). *The Retinal Atlas*, 2nd edn. Elsevier, Oxford.

# The screening episode: visual acuity, mydriasis, and digital photography

David K. Roy and Prashant Amrelia

> **KEY POINTS**
>
> - This chapter will review the screening episode, measuring visual acuity, drop instillation, contraindications, and correct camera operation.
> - It will review problems associated with incorrect camera operation and the NHS Diabetic Eye Screening Programme (NHSDESP) standards of acceptable image quality.
> - This will guide the screener in obtaining clear, well-centred, gradable digital images of the retina, as well as providing a greater understanding of the issues associated with screening

The screening episode is of paramount importance. The detection and accurate diagnosis of diabetic retinopathy (DR) and timely referral for treatment is only possible if optimum quality images are captured to NHSDESP national standards.

## 10.1  Measuring visual acuity/drop instillation

### 10.1.1  Visual 'acuity'

Visual 'acuity' (VA) is derived from the Latin word 'acuitas' (sharpness). It is used to describe the smallest letters that can be read without refractive correction on a visual acuity chart.

A common method for measuring visual acuity is using the Snellen chart (see Figure 10.1), devised by a Dutch ophthalmologist, Dr Herman Snellen, in 1892. The chart consists of lines of printed block letters. The first line consists of the largest letter, which may be one of several letters, followed by rows of letters decreasing in size.

The person taking the test covers one eye, often with an occluder and reads aloud the letters of each row, starting from the top. The smallest letter row that

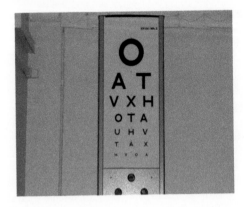

Figure 10.1 Snellen chart.
Reproduced courtesy of Professor Paul M. Dodson and The Heart of England Retinal Screening Centre.

can be read accurately indicates the patient's visual acuity in that eye and is recorded. More recently, health-care professionals have introduced the LogMAR chart (logarithm of the minimum angle of resolution; see Figure 10.2), following recommendations of the American National Academy of Sciences National Research Council. The LogMAR method has been found to be more accurate and reproducible than the Snellen method, and is being introduced into routine clinical practice, particularly for paediatrics and acuity measurements for research, to improve accuracy.

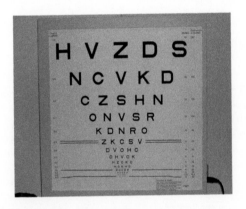

Figure 10.2 LogMAR chart.
Reproduced courtesy of Professor Paul M. Dodson and The Heart of England Retinal Screening Centre.

## 10.2 Visual acuity testing during a screening episode

### 10.2.1 The importance of visual acuity testing

VA is a most important measurement of visual function and should be measured with the patient wearing their glasses to correct any known refractive error. Alternatively, a simple pinhole device can be used, either by itself or in combination with glasses. The pinhole device (occluder) only allows light rays through the principal axis to the retina, thus minimizing refractive errors of the cornea and lens, and therefore providing a measure of best corrected vision. At every screening episode patients with diabetes should have their VA measured and recorded on the screening software, as it is integral to the clinical outcome, e.g. the referable maculopathy definition outlined in Chapter 6, 'Maculopathy'.

Visual acuity is best measured using the 6-m method (a patient sitting 6 m away from the Snellen chart), which may be set up using mirrors in small rooms, e.g. two 3-m distances.

Adapted Snellen charts are also available with the same apparent letter size to the person at shorter distances of 3 m.

Normal VA is around the 6/6 (6/4 to 6/9) level, but may vary, particularly with lighting level, refractive error, amblyopia, and variable glucose control.

Where previous screening information and VA is available, it is a useful comparison to assess change, which could indicate ocular disease.

Following measurement of the VA, the retinal screener should check the nature and timings of visual loss, as well as previous, ocular interventions, and record the details. For example, uni-ocular poor vision may be the result of amblyopia, commonly as a result of a squint in childhood. Not taking an appropriate visual history may result in unnecessary referrals to ophthalmology clinics.

To measure *visual acuity*:

- Position the patient directly facing the VA chart.
- Start with the right eye, first occluding the left eye.
- If glasses or lenses are worn for distance vision, ensure the patient is wearing them.
- Record how vision was measured, i.e. unaided, with glasses, or with pinhole.
- VA is measured by distance and size of letters, e.g. 6/12.
  - Top figure 6 = distance in metres between patient and chart.
  - Bottom figure 12 = the last complete line the patient can read.
- If the patient is unable to read the top line at 6 m (6/60), take them to a 3-m distance and measure as before. This alters readings to 3/60.
- If still unable to read top letter at 3 m then:
  - a recording of count fingers (CF) is made by holding two or three fingers at a distance of 1 m; or

    ○ a recording of hand movements (HM) by holding your hand about 1 m away and gently waving hand;

    ○ the next level is perception of light (PL) or no perception of light (NPL) (note that there are differences in screening programmes as to the protocol for whether to screen PL or NPL eyes, but recent data suggest that digital photography is not worthwhile).

- Repeat VA recording for the other eye.

## Drop instillation ensuring mydriasis

- Check that visual acuity has already been tested and recorded.

- Patients must be warned prior to a screening visit by letter *not to drive* for 4–6 hours afterwards. This must be clearly stipulated in patient information leaflets or invitation letters.

- *Always* check allergy status before instilling any drops into the eyes; if unsure seek advice.

- Ensure correct patient identification (ask the patient for their date of birth, address, or other identifiers if unsure).

- Ensure local infection-control hand-washing procedure is followed.

- Make sure drops have been stored appropriately and are within the use-by date.

- Topical tropicamide, 1% solution at 1 drop, is the common dilating agent used. Apply drops to the fornix, which will ensure that the agent is maximally absorbed.

- A minimum of 20 minutes is required for adequate pupil dilatation.

- If there is insufficient pupil dilatation with 1 drop of 1% tropicamide as described above, a repeat of 1% tropicamide in addition to phenylephrine 2.5% should be instilled.

## 10.4 Contraindications to pupil dilatation

### 10.4.1 Dilating patients with glaucoma?

The concern and contraindication of pharmacological pupil dilatation in patients with glaucoma has become embedded in medicine. The concern arises from the risk of precipitation of acute glaucoma in patients with a narrow anterior chamber angle. This is a very rare event, and should not occur in patients with known glaucoma as appropriate treatment (e.g. iridotomy for closed-angle glaucoma) will have been performed, thereby making pupil dilatation safe. The common open-angle glaucoma can be dilated safely. However, patients should be warned in patient information leaflets that, if they develop the suggestive symptoms of acute glaucoma including acute pain and a red eye, hours after mydriasis, they should report urgently to a hospital eye casualty department.

### 10.4.2 Iris clip lens

Up to 1984, an intra-ocular lens implant used following cataract extraction was an iris clip lens, placed in the anterior chamber of the eye (see Figure 10.3). This lens was held in place by studs on the pupil surface, such that pupil dilatation would result in anterior dislocation of the prosthetic lens. This would result in a dissatisfied patient, because of visual distortion and the requirement for further ocular surgery. The presence of this type of lens can be detected by anterior chamber photography as in Figure 10.3, and is an absolute contraindication to mydriasis.

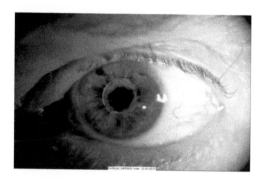

Figure 10.3 **An iris clip lens.**
Reproduced courtesy of Professor Paul M. Dodson and The Heart of England Retinal Screening Centre.

### 10.4.3 Patient group directive

As of 2007 in the UK, an essential advance has been to allow retinal screeners to perform visual acuity and mydriasis without medical supervision, providing screening staff have completed the appropriate certified training and competencies. Most hospitals and screening programmes will have protocols for a patient group directive (PGD) agreement to instil mydriatic drops without a doctor's signed prescription each time. It may be a preprinted prescription allowing staff to check visual acuity and to instil dilating drops using a standard protocol, stressing safe practice with appropriate exclusions and advice about not driving following mydriasis.

## 10.5 Taking acceptable digital retinal images

A retinal screener's role is to obtain the best possible images, as well as gathering and recording correct information during the photography session. It is imperative to ascertain whether the patient is already under hospital diabetic eye services, as screening may not be appropriate (i.e. the patient, by definition, has a referable disease).

- *Position the patient comfortably*: ask the patient to rest their chin on the rest and forehead on the bar, correctly aligning the patient's eyes with the camera alignment markers (see Figure 10.4).

Incorrect alignment                    Correct alignment

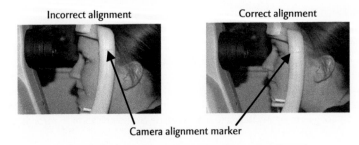

Camera alignment marker

Figure 10.4 **Eye alignments with the camera lens.**
Reproduced courtesy of Professor Paul M. Dodson and The Heart of England Retinal Screening Centre.

- *Explain what they will experience, e.g. a bright flash*: ask the patient to follow the internal or external fixation light.
- Move camera sliding base forward, returning the camera mirror control (a button on the top of the sliding camera base) until the retina is clearly visible. Adjust the focusing control and joystick until the correct field is obtained.

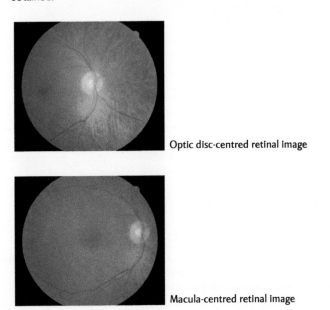

Optic disc-centred retinal image

Macula-centred retinal image

Figure 10.5 **The two standard views obtained,** (top) one centred on the optic disc and (bottom) the other on the macula.
Reproduced courtesy of Professor Paul M. Dodson and The Heart of England Retinal Screening Centre.

- Take a macula-centred and optic disc-centred view for each eye (see Figure 10.5). This is standard for the NHSDESP, but there are variations in other programmes, e.g. using a single macula view only.

### 10.5.1 Should one or two retinal images be captured?

While two fields of view digital retinal photography (one macula-centred and one optic disc-centred) is the accepted method of screening in the English national programme, achieving high sensitivity (>80%) and specificity (>90%), it has been argued by some authorities that only one macula-centred image is necessary. Adoption of the latter cuts down screening time and costs, as well as reducing server storage-space requirements. A recent study investigated whether there is any benefit in doing the optic disc view in addition to just the macula-centred view. This demonstrated that obtaining a macula-centred view alone compared with the two views missed one in five cases of proliferative retinopathy, and two in five of cases with pre-proliferative DR and there is, therefore, a concern that clinical outcomes would be altered. These data support the principle that two fields of view are superior in accuracy for identification of levels of DR, as in the English programme.

Other settings will be needed for illumination and camera flash, which will be specified by camera manufacturers.

### 10.5.2 Anterior chamber photography

If the retinal view is hazy, it is useful to photograph an anterior chamber view. To do this:

- Using the camera compensation filters (magnification lens diopters to adjust for + or − normal refractive changes), pull control fully out.
- Adjust so that the front of the eye (anterior chamber) is showing on the camera monitor.
- Focus on the pupil (set to fine focus, thus sharpening the image).
- Take the photograph.

Examples of the value of anterior chamber photographs are shown in Chapter 4, 'Diabetes and the eye', and Chapter 17, 'Patients of concern', for example demonstrating the different types of cataracts.

## 10.6 Problems with digital fundal photography

### 10.6.1 Camera operational problems you *can* control

- *Dark photos*: often due to poor pupil dilatation; increase the flash level or leave for longer dilatation. May need more mydriatics (see Figure 10.6).
- *Rim artefact*: check patient's head is resting on the chin rest facing squarely straight ahead (see Figure 10.7).

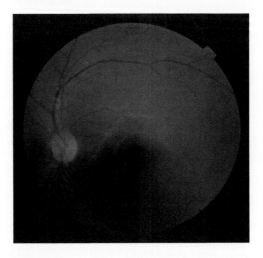

Figure 10.6 **Dark photo.**
Reproduced courtesy of Professor Paul M. Dodson and The Heart of England Retinal Screening Centre.

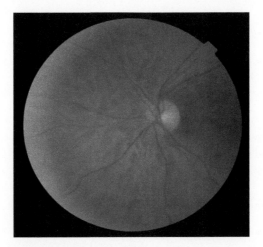

Figure 10.7 'Rim artefact'. Artefact around the periphery.
Reproduced courtesy of Professor Paul M. Dodson and The Heart of England Retinal Screening Centre.

### 10.6.1.1 *Circle photographic artefact*

Pull camera out and reposition if the camera alignment is incorrect, with the camera being either too close, too far away, or not over the centre of the retina.

## 10.6.2 Problems you *can't* control

- Cataracts may result in an ungradable digital image, which will require referral for slit lamp biomicroscopy examination (see Chapter 3, Figure 3.1).
- *Asteroid hyalosis*: these are particles in the vitreous due to calcium soaps and commonly result in ungradable photographs (see Figure 10.8). It may be difficult to distinguish if the opacities in the vitreous are asteroid particles or exudates as they can look identical in appearance. Patients may need to have retinal screening performed long-term by slit lamp biomicroscopy examination.

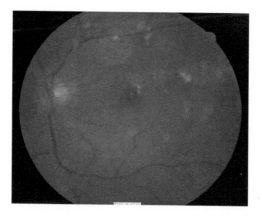

Figure 10.8 **Asteroid hyalosis.**
Reproduced courtesy of Professor Paul M. Dodson and The Heart of England Retinal Screening Centre.

- *Artefacts on the camera lens*: marks on the camera lens may cause artefacts that may compromise the fundal image area, making the image difficult to grade, or may be mistaken for retinal pathology (see Figure 10.9). Other small dots and black artefacts may appear on an image, which may be caused by dust settling on the camera chip due to static build-up. This will probably require specialist help from the camera suppliers.

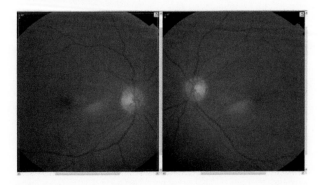

Figure 10.9 A lens artefact, which is clear as it occupies the same position in the photograph regardless of centring.

Reproduced courtesy of Professor Paul M. Dodson and The Heart of England Retinal Screening Centre.

## 10.7 NHSDESP standards/targets of acceptable image quality

- 2 × nominal 45-degree fields per eye (see Figure 10.5).
- A macula-centred view field is taken so that any maculopathy can be clearly detected, and a disc (nasal) view can assist with detecting pre-proliferative retinopathy in the periphery of the retina (R2) and proliferative retinopathy (R3).
- Taking two views helps with detecting artefacts that disappear or move on one of the two views taken.
- Images should only be utilized if the grader is confident about the quality of the screening photographs.
- All grading must be performed by trained and accredited staff (see Chapter 11, 'How to grade', and Chapter 15, 'Training and accreditation for retinal screening and grading').
- Inadequate (ungradable) images are those that fail to meet the definition of adequate as described above.

FURTHER READING

Gov.UK. (2014). Diabetic eye screening: programme overview. An overview of the NHS diabetic eye screening (DES) programme, its services and contact information. https://www.gov.uk/guidance/diabetic-eye-screening-programme-overview (accessed 20 August 2019).

Public Health England. (2019). PHE screening: NHS Diabetic Eye Screening Programme. https://phescreening.blog.gov.uk/category/des/ (accessed 20 August 2019).

Shah M, Fellows H, Wharton H, Quant L, Dodson PM. (2017). One field of view versus two fields of view: is a macula centred photograph adequate for diabetic retinopathy screening? *Int J Ophthal Vision Res* **1**(1): 001–5.

Wharton H, Cash K, Hazelgrove K, Mills A, Jacobs S, Dodson PM. (2019). Should we photograph eyes with perception of light (NPL) during diabetic eye screening? *Eur J Ophthal* **29**(3): NP12–NP36.

CHAPTER 10

# CHAPTER 11

# How to grade

Karen Whitehouse

---

**KEY POINTS**

- This chapter will provide guidance on best practice.
- A good grader should have the ability to work autonomously and have a keen attention to detail; the grading environment should be quiet with appropriate lighting and grading should be undertaken on high quality computer equipment and screens.
- All graders will adopt their own methodology for grading and use a step-by-step method, which may also use image manipulation.
- For accuracy and consistency, graders should adhere to minimum standards and numbers of grades as required by the NHS Diabetic Eye Screening Programme (NHSDESP).
- In the UK, graders should be adequately trained, and participate in monthly test and training sets.

---

## 11.1 The grading environment

The environment that a grader works in is very important in order to ensure that grading is consistently accurate. The equipment that a grader requires cannot be compromised and the room should be adequately darkened, preventing any glare on the computer screen, which may interfere with their view of images. The room should be as quiet as possible, with distractions kept to a minimum, helping to minimize human error. Where possible, graders should be working in close proximity to other competent graders who can give advice—helping to increase a grader's confidence—and allowing a team to learn from one another (see Figure 11.1).

## 11.2 The job role of a grader

An optimum workload for a grader, together with the necessary training and maintenance of expertise, is essential to maintain skills, grading accuracy, and job satisfaction.

The NHSDESP states that programmes should monitor the number of image sets graded in a session, in the context of the individual grader's intergrader agreement report, in order to ensure that the speed of grading does not affect

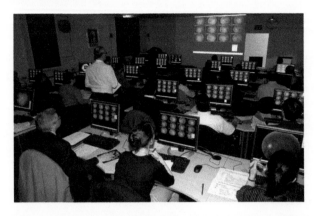

Figure 11.1 An example of an open-plan grading laboratory. (The grading and training facility at Heartlands Hospital Screening Centre.)

Reproduced courtesy of Professor Paul M. Dodson and The Heart of England Retinal Screening Centre.

quality. Arbitration and referral outcome grading may require additional grading time due to the more complex choice of patient outcomes and reporting.

One of the key objectives of a screening scheme is to have a high sensitivity and specificity, thereby preventing false positives (unnecessary referrals) and false negatives (non-referral of referable images). The accuracy of grading is fundamental to this and is a key factor for a screening programme achieving a satisfactory external quality assessment (peer review) report.

In the UK, graders who do not hold additional job roles as either an optometrist or an ophthalmologist must grade a minimum of 1000 patient image sets per annum.

Graders who also are qualified optometrists and undertake this job role, and do not grade 1000 image sets must grade a minimum of 500 image sets, and then supplement this number with 10 image sets from the online test and training set.

If an optometrist grader does not grade the minimum number of image sets, then evidence of participation in the online test and training set should be provided.

### 11.2.1 Non-grading photographers

Non-grading photographers (screeners) must still have sufficient skills in order to triage the patient accurately. It is mandatory that they undertake appropriate training and supervision, in order to take excellent, relevant images and triage appropriately in order to accelerate image grading where necessary. It is also crucial that a relevant visual history is taken in order for the grader and referral outcome grader (ROG) to come to a correct clinical outcome.

## 11.3 How to grade

### 11.3.1 National grading standards

The local grading protocols of all diabetic eye screening programmes within England must abide by the English Retinopathy Grading Classification devised by the NHSDESP. This is due to the need to assess programme performance against the set criteria during audit, and allow assessment of the national programme as a whole.

Small, local referral variations may apply at the discretion of the clinical lead, but are generally additions in grades or subdivisions of the grading criteria.

Each eye photographed should receive a retinopathy 'R grade' and a maculopathy 'M grade'.

Note: graders should regularly refer to national guidelines for any updates to classification.

### 11.3.2 Retinopathy grading: 'The R grade'

The R grade indicates the level of retinopathy for the whole retinal image in question.

#### 11.3.2.1 R0 (none)

- No visible diabetic retinopathy (DR) on images.

#### 11.3.2.2 R1 (background diabetic retinopathy)

- Microaneurysm(s).
- Retinal haemorrhages.
- Venous loop.
- Any exudate in the presence of other non-referable features of DR.
- Any number of cotton wool spots (CWS) in the presence of other non-referable features of DR.

#### 11.3.2.3 R2 (pre-proliferative diabetic retinopathy)

- Venous beading.
- Venous reduplication.
- Multiple blot haemorrhages.
- Intra-retinal microvascular abnormality (IRMA).

#### 11.3.2.4 R3 (proliferative diabetic retinopathy)

Active proliferative retinopathy:
- New vessels elsewhere (NVE).
- New vessels on the disc (NVD).
- Pre-retinal haemorrhage.

- Vitreous haemorrhage.
- Pre-retinal fibrosis +/− tractional retinal detachment.
- Reactivation in a previous stable R3S eye.

### 11.3.3 Maculopathy grading: 'The M grade'

#### 11.3.3.1 *Definition of the macula*

The NHSDESP currently defines the macula as that part of the retina that lies within a circle centred on the centre of the fovea, whose radius is the distance between the centre of the fovea and the temporal margin of the disc. Software may allow the grader to apply a grid that will assist in the measurement of any pathology within the macular region.

The M grade indicates the amount of DR within the critical macular region of the eye.

#### 11.3.3.2 *M0 (no maculopathy)*

Absence of any M1 features: no exudates or haemorrhages within the macular region.

#### 11.3.3.3 *M1 (referable maculopathy)*

An eye should be graded as M1 if there is:

- exudate within one disc diameter (DD) of the centre of the fovea; *or*
- a group of exudates within the macula—revised grading classification for groups of exudates:
  - A group of exudates is an area of exudates that is greater than or equal to half the disc area and this area (of greater than or equal to half the disc area) is all within the macular area.
  - The outer points of the exudates are joined and compared with half the area of the optic disc; *or*
- any microaneurysm or haemorrhage within 1DD of the centre of the fovea, only if associated with a best visual acuity (VA) of 6/12 or worse (0.3 LogMAR).

If there is any maculopathy present, then the R grade must be a minimum of R1 (as this means that there is a minimum of background retinopathy on the whole retina).

### 11.3.4 Patient outcomes from grading

See Table 11.1.

**Table 11.1** Patient outcomes from grading

| DR grade | Outcome |
|---|---|
| R0M0 (No DR present) | Annual recall |
| R1M0 (Background no maculopathy) | Annual recall |
| R2M0 (Pre-proliferative + no maculopathy) | Routine referral to HES/DS |
| R1M1 (Maculopathy) | Routine referral to HES/DS |
| R2M1 (Pre-proliferative and maculopathy) | Routine referral to HES/DS |
| R3M0 (Proliferative + no maculopathy) | *Urgent* referral to HES |
| R3M1 (Proliferative + maculopathy) | *Urgent* referral to HES |
| U (Ungradable image) | Routine referral to HES or slit lamp biomicroscopy (SLB) |
| Other lesions | Referred as per local protocols |

HES, hospital eye service; DS, digital surveillance.

This service operates as an interim to referral and may incorporate optical coherence tomography to monitor the patient; programmes will have different referral criteria for their patients and so the grader should be *au fait* with the agreed local criteria and pathway.

## 11.3.5 Other gradings

### 11.3.5.1 *Presence of laser*

Patients who are graded as R3S following discharge from the hospital eye service (HES) may be managed in the digital surveillance (DS) pathway.

Patients with stable treated retinopathy, currently in routine annual screening, should be graded as R3S at their next routine annual screen, and have benchmark images taken and transferred to the DS pathway, for their next and subsequent routine appointments.

- *Presence of laser treatment for new vessels* (laser around periphery—known as pan-retinal photocoagulation): the grade is always R3, along with a P (photocoagulation) plus the M grade as per any other grade. If there is no *new* neovascularization or fibrosis then this should be graded as R3S(P) 'stable treated proliferative diabetic retinopathy' and put on 12 months DS recall, if no other referable pathology is present.

- *Presence of laser treatment for maculopathy* (laser around macula). This should be graded as P, but the M grade should be assessed on the current status of the macula, e.g. R1M0(P).

## 11.4 Image quality

Two 45-degree fields of each eye should be captured—a foveal-centred and a disc-centred view—and the grading should take into account both of these views, together with an assessment of both the position and image quality (clarity) of each field. The quality of an image can be classed as either adequate or inadequate (i.e. ungradable).

### 11.4.1 Adequate view macular-centred image

#### 11.4.1.1 *Position*

The centre of the fovea should be within or 1DD from the centre of the image (see Figure 11.2).

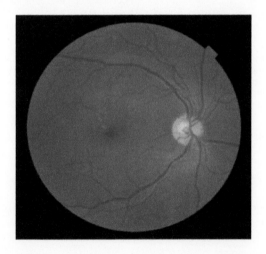

Figure 11.2 A macular view classed as 'adequate'. Note exudate encroaching on the fovea.
Reproduced courtesy of Professor Paul M. Dodson and The Heart of England Retinal Screening Centre.

#### 11.4.1.2 *Clarity*

Vessels should be clearly visible within 1DD of the centre of the fovea.

## 11.4.2 Adequate view disc-centred image

### 11.4.2.1 *Position*

The centre of the disc should be within 1DD of the centre of the image (see Figure 11.3).

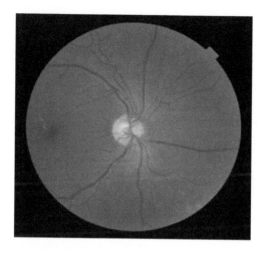

Figure 11.3 **A disc-centred view classed as 'adequate'.**

Reproduced courtesy of Professor Paul M. Dodson and The Heart of England Retinal Screening Centre.

### 11.4.2.2 *Clarity*

Vessels should be clearly visible on the surface of the disc.

Failure to meet the standards of an adequate view results in it being graded as inadequate (U) and the patient referred as routine to the HES or slit lamp biomicroscopy (SLB) service. The exception to this is if *referable retinopathy is visible anywhere on the image* (R2, R3, M1, unstable treated retinopathy).

Dependent upon the level of pathology, the patient should be referred to the HES or SLB service to obtain a grade for patients who are not assessable by digital photography.

The national standard deemed acceptable where the 'proportion of eligible people with diabetes where a digital image has been obtained, but the final grading outcome is ungradable' is 2–4%.

Ungradable (U) images can be classified in the following way:

• Unable to image because of person-specific factors.
• Digital image possible in one eye, but ungradable in second eye.

- Ungradable in both eyes, due to a condition amenable to treatment.
- Ungradable in both eyes, due to a condition amenable to treatment, but for which treatment is not yet indicated.
- Ungradable in both eyes, due to a condition not amenable to treatment, but possible to visualize the retina using SLB.
- Ungradable in both eyes and not possible to visualize the retina with any other method.

The percentage of ungradable images will vary from scheme to scheme, depending upon the incidence of cataracts and other lesions in populations, and this should be taken into account.

## 11.5 Image manipulation

Using digital photography to screen patients allows a host of image manipulation tools to enhance the quality of the images. Graders should use these to grade an image before grading it as not assessable.

However, brightening-up and over-manipulation can cause an image to become grainy and more difficult to grade. In addition, the pale areas, such as the disc, may become too light. It is good practice to assess an image in colour without any manipulation first.

Using red-free manipulation can be useful, as it reveals vascular pathology more clearly. It is particularly useful in the diagnosis of IRMA and new vessels on an image, which may be less clear on a colour image (Figure 11.4).

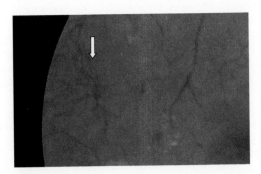

Figure 11.4 This red-free enhanced view demonstrates NVE. The arrow shows the area of new vessels.

### 11.5.1 Step-by-step guide to grading

Every grader will have their own method for grading; here, a step-by-step guide is suggested to ensure that every part of the retina is checked and graded sufficiently.

1. *Check visual acuities*: this may affect the grade/outcome.
2. *Assess the whole image*:
   ○ What is the image quality?
   ○ Is the image assessable?
3. Look at the rest of the retina and vasculature on the macular view and assess for R grade (retinopathy) or any other lesions.
   Take particular care when viewing the periphery.
   ○ Either R0, R1, R2, or R3.
4. Enlarge the *macular-centred view* and magnify the macula to assess for the M grade (maculopathy): either M0 or M1.
5. Look at the retina on the *optic disc view* and assess for R (retinopathy) grade or any other lesions, and confirm the M grade (may identify artefacts as these can alter between the two images).
   Take particular care when viewing the periphery.
6. Magnify the optic disc, and assess for any DR or other lesions.
7. *View any previous images*: compare any abnormalities/assess changes.
8. View anterior chamber pictures if available.
9. Medical history:
   ○ Look for any HES appointments, e.g. has the patient been discharged, have they been lost to follow-up, or have they not attended previous HES appointments?
   ○ Check for any comments about medical or ophthalmic history.
10. Input the grade +/− comments into the software and do the same with the other eye.

While this schema is only a rough guide, lesions will be missed if a system is not employed by each individual and appropriate time not spent on each set of images.

## 11.6 Image quality

Programmes report on intergrader disagreements in order to assess quality of their grading, which may identify grader issues that may need to be evaluated.

Any graders who are identified as causing higher levels of arbitration or whose intergrader agreement (percentage agreement with the final outcome grade) demonstrates that there are significant differences in grading outcomes compared with the final grade by senior graders, may therefore require further training or supervision.

## 11.7 Test and training

The online (DRS EQA) test and training system supports programmes to quality-assure graders and to measure performance. These should be assessed in conjunction with local grader performance reports within their programme to assess how the grader is performing. It is also a valuable tool to provide training sets for new staff.

A minimum of 10 sets per annum should be completed by each grader, but it is good practice to try and complete the test sets each month, as this will help graders evaluate how they are grading in relation to national grading criteria.

## 11.8 Health screener qualification

The Health Screener Diploma (level 3) has been introduced for health screeners (diabetic eye, abdominal aortic aneurysm, and newborn hearing screening programmes) and is appropriate for screeners, graders, and screener/graders. It involves mandatory units, which all screeners complete, and role-specific units to ensure competence, knowledge, and ability are all confirmed (see Chapter 15, 'Training and accreditation for retinal screening and grading').

FURTHER READING

Gov.UK. (2012). Diabetic eye screening: retinal image grading criteria. https://www.gov.uk/government/publications/diabetic-eye-screening-retinal-image-grading-criteria (accessed 20 August 2019).

Gov.UK. (2014). Diabetic eye screening programme: pathway standards. https://www.gov.uk/government/publications/diabetic-eye-screening-standards-and-performance-objectives (accessed 20 August 2019).

NHS Screening Programmes. (2016). The management of grading quality: good practice in the quality assurance of grading. https://assets.publishing.service.gov.uk/government/uploads/system/uploads/attachment_data/file/512832/The_Management_of_Grading.pdf (accessed 20 August 2019).

Public Health England. (2017). NHS Diabetic Eye Screening Programme: grading definitions for referable disease. https://assets.publishing.service.gov.uk/government/uploads/system/uploads/attachment_data/file/582710/Grading_definitions_for_referrable_disease_2017_new_110117.pdf (accessed 20 August 2019).

Scanlon PH, Malhotra R, Thomas G, Foy C, Kirkpatrick JN, Lewis-Barned N, et al. (2003). The effectiveness of screening for diabetic retinopathy by digital imaging photography and technician ophthalmoscopy. *Diabet Med* **20**(6): 467–74. https://www.ncbi.nlm.nih.gov/pubmed/12786681 (accessed 22 November 2019).

# CHAPTER 12

# The principles of a national diabetic eye screening programme

Paul Galsworthy

**KEY POINTS**

- The aim of the programme is to reduce the risk of sight loss by prompt identification and effective treatment.
- Screening programmes consist of various key components to manage patients through the pathway.
- Who to screen and how frequently.
- Screening models/modes.
- Screening pathway and standards.

## 12.1 Introduction

Diabetic eye screening programmes (DESPs) are in place in many countries across the world, with an aim to reduce the risk of sight loss among people with diabetes by the prompt identification and effective treatment of sight-threatening retinopathy at the appropriate stage during the disease process.

A diabetic retinopathy (DR) screening programme should consist of several key components:

- Programme management.
- Clinical leadership.
- Administration of the programme to:
    - systematically identify the cohort of all diabetics in a population;
    - invite the cohort to screening;
    - report outcomes.
- Screening test (digital image capture).
- Grading of digital images.
- The surveillance pathway using:
    - slit lamp biomicroscopy (SLB clinics);
    - digital image surveillance (DS clinics).
- Ophthalmology referral (diagnosis, treatment, and outcomes).
- Fail-safe, so subjects do not get lost to care systems.
- Internal quality assurance (IQA) and programme reporting.

It is important for all DESPs to ensure the following roles are fulfilled:

- Clinical lead and/or ophthalmology lead.
- Programme manager.
- Senior screener/graders.
- Screener/graders.
- Fail-safe officers.
- Administrators.

## 12.2 Who to screen and frequency of screening

At present, the eligible population for diabetic eye screening is all people with Type 1 or Type 2 diabetes, aged 12 years and over, who have light perception or better in at least one eye, unless they have been excluded or suspended according to national guidance. These have been laid out in national documents on the NHSDESP website entitled 'Exclusions, suspensions and management of ungradables'. Not all eligible patients are offered screening, for example people who are under the care of the hospital eye service (HES) for diabetic eye disease are not invited for annual eye screening, although it is important that fail-safe measures are in place to ensure this cohort of patients are being seen in HES and the results are being fed back to the programme (see Chapter 13, 'Programme administration and fail-safe') so that subjects do not get lost within the pathway.

There have been studies that have confirmed that 12 years of age is the right age to start screening, as no patients have been identified with sight-threatening DR under this age, but patients were identified with background DR under the age 12. The decision of whether to screen for life, once diabetes is established, needs to be studied in diabetic populations. The author's recent data suggested that there was little benefit of screening 90-year-old subjects and older, as no serious DR was identified, but referrals were appropriate for other lesions, e.g. cataracts.

Multiple studies have now confirmed that lower risk patients do not need to be screened on an annual basis as the risk of development of sight-threatening DR within a 2-year period is low. In line with a number of other countries, the UK national screening committee has recommended implementing 2-year (extended screening) intervals. This is likely to be implemented using a phased approach, and programmes in the UK should start to look into the implementation of such a change by reviewing their grading quality, capacity, staffing, patient engagement/communication, and commissioning implications. A number of countries have already implemented extended screening intervals for those patients with no DR in either eye, with some countries adopting a longer screening interval than every 2 years. An alternative approach is to assess individual subjects' risk of development of DR using demographic and clinical data in a computerized risk engine similar to that used in cardiovascular risk prediction (e.g. Framingham equation). However, to adopt this approach, the screening programme needs access to patients' clinical data, usually from primary care. While this approach is in place, research into large programmes is ongoing to validate these systems.

Low-risk patients have been defined as having no DR in either eye on two consecutive screening episodes. Subjects with any background (R1) DR are to continue to be screened annually in the UK programme.

It is also important to note that patients who have had various surgical interventions, such as weight loss (bariatric) surgery or pancreatic transplant (see Chapter 16, 'Medical management of diabetic retinopathy') to try to achieve a 'cure' for their diabetes, continue to be screened under current guidance. These patients are classed as 'diabetes in remission' and not 'resolved'.

## 12.3 Screening programme models

All screening programmes should cover at least 12,000 people with diabetes (i.e. serving a general population of approximately 500,000). Programmes need to be sufficiently large to enable meaningful comparable data to be collected and to ensure enough exposure of images to enable expertise amongst graders.

There are two main screening models that have been adopted around the UK, although some programmes adopt a combination of the two.

### 12.3.1 Mobile

Screening is undertaken for set periods of time at a range of locations, such as GP surgeries and community centres, by transporting screening equipment to alternating locations. Alternatively, screening is actually undertaken within a customized mobile screening van.

### 12.3.2 Fixed optometry

Screening is undertaken at specific local programme-accredited optometry practices. Screening equipment does not move and screening is available all year round at each location.

There are two call/recall models used—open and closed invitation.

### 12.3.3 Open invitation

This requires the patient to contact the local eye screening programme following receipt of their invitation. Patients can either call a central administration team or can call their desired screening site (optometry model) to book an appointment that meets their circumstances.

### 12.3.4 Closed invitation

Patients are offered a pre-booked appointment (often at their own GP or preferred location). An administration team is still required for patients wishing to amend their appointment.

Some programmes may operate a mixed model having some locations/areas with open and closed type of invitations. Both models have their advantages and disadvantages—programmes should operate a recall model that suits their screening model, demographics, and geography of the catchment area. In the UK, the majority of schemes are of the mobile type, with fixed screening invitation.

Prior to the common pathway being introduced in 2013 there were many inconsistencies among diabetic eye screening programmes, including variations with grading and subsequent referral pathways. This had financial and reporting implications, i.e. how funding was distributed between screening programmes for diagnosis and HES for treatment, and difficulties in obtaining consistency between programmes, and hence, an accurate national report and assessment.

The common pathway defined new pathways, redefined grading criteria, and introduced feature-based grading. It also clarified suspension and exclusion criteria, and introduced the digital surveillance (DS) pathway, which provided screening for patients requiring more frequent, flexible interval screening out of routine annual digital screening (RDS). This group of patients in the DS pathway are managed and reported separately to those on RDS.

## 12.4 The surveillance pathway

DS clinics have been incorporated into the screening programme, as it was clear that many referable maculopathy patients (M1) had early lesions, and these could be more closely monitored and managed in a virtual system. Final grading for this pathway is completed by referral outcome graders and patients who are either discharged if changes resolve or referred into ophthalmology services if their condition deteriorates and macular oedema develops. Since optical coherence tomography (OCT) is an integral part in the diagnosis and management of macular oedema, it has become increasingly popular to incorporate this into DS clinics and is a logical progression for patient care.

The DS pathway also has been recommended for monitoring of pre-proliferative DR and those with stable proliferative DR, who can be safely discharged from eye clinics to be monitored within the screening programme.

### 12.4.1 Digital surveillance is made of two clinics and pathways

Digital photographic surveillance clinics are suitable for the closer monitoring of patients with eye disease who do not require treatment in the HES. DS clinics are also used for the more frequent screening of pregnant patients throughout their pregnancy, and patients of concern, as described in Chapter 16, 'Medical management of diabetic retinopathy'.

Slit lamp biomicroscopy (SLB) clinics serve the other group of patients who have unassessable images (where fundus images do not permit accurate grading), e.g. with cataracts or asteroid hyalosis, who can be screened within an SLB clinic and adequate views obtained.

Regardless of the delivery model or invitation process, all programmes should follow the diabetic eye screening (DES) patient pathway as illustrated in Figure 12.1.

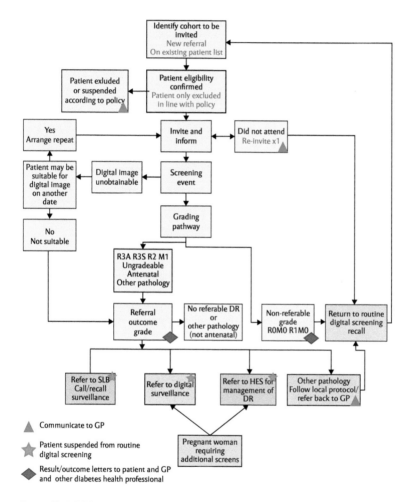

Figure 12.1 DES patient pathway.

The DES patient pathway and screening standards encompass the entire screening pathway and are based on the following themes:

- accurate identification of the diabetic population;
- informing the population for screening;
- maximum coverage and/or uptake;
- accurate screening test;
- correct diagnosis and appropriate quality assurance;
- appropriate intervention/treatment in a timely manner;
- minimizing harm;
- ensuring appropriate staff training and education;
- ensuring robust commissioning and governance.

## 12.5 Quality assurance

The purpose of quality assurance (QA) is to:

- Reduce the probability of error.
- Ensure that errors are dealt with competently and sensitively.
- Help professional and organization improvement year-on-year.
- Set and re-set standards (national responsibility).

It is important that all screening programmes follow national QA standards in order to ensure the service is safe and effective. There are various standards and key performance indicators (KPIs) that are used to measure a programme; these data can be used to compare one programme to another, and can be assessed as a whole national programme.

### 12.5.1 Service specification (Service specification 22)

This has been provided to ensure a consistent and equitable approach across the country, and to govern the provision and monitoring of the NHSDESP. The service specification outlines the service and quality indicators expected by NHS England (NHSE). This is available on the Internet at www.gov.uk (search for 'Commissioning public health').

## 12.6 Key performance indicators

In the UK, KPIs are reported quarterly and focus on key areas of particular concern, and often, when a KPI consistently reaches the achievable level, it becomes a standard.

The DESP in the UK currently has three KPIs:

- *DE1*: percentage uptake of routine digital screening event.
- *DE2*: to achieve all results of screening being issued within 3 weeks of RDS, digital surveillance, or slit lamp biomicroscopy attendances.
- *DE3*: timely assessment for those identified with active proliferative retinopathy (i.e. to ensure urgent appointments are achieved).

KPIs are a useful tool to assess the really important key outcomes of screening programmes. While the three given above are used in the UK programme, it is clear that these will differ in other countries.

## 12.7 Diabetic eye screening pathway standards in the UK

The national programme has developed pathway standards in joint collaboration with experts in relevant fields, using available evidence, data, and best practice. The purpose of such standards are to collect reliable and timely information, regarding the quality standards from all screening programmes. Data can be reviewed at a local, regional, and national level, resulting in a consistent approach to screening delivery. Experience from other national programmes has shown variation in these standards that is more appropriate to their method of screening and health service delivery.

As of April 2017, the standards have been revised for the diabetic eye; there are now 13 standards, which are listed in Table 12.1.

**Table 12.1** Summary of diabetic eye screening programme standards

| Standard | Objective | Description | Thresholds |
|---|---|---|---|
| DES-PS1 | To maximize the proportion of all known eligible people with diabetes who are invited to attend for routine digital screening and to monitor the proportion of the eligible population who are suspended or excluded | 1.1 Percentage of eligible people, categorized under RDS, who are offered an appointment for RDS | Acceptable: ≥95% Achievable: ≥98% |
| | | 1.2 Percentage of eligible people, categorized as suspended | To be set |
| | | 1.3 Percentage of eligible people, categorized as excluded | To be set |
| DES-PS2 | To invite all people newly diagnosed with diabetes to attend for routine DR screening | Proportion of people newly diagnosed with diabetes offered a first RDS appointment that is due to occur within 89 calendar days of the provider being notified of their diagnosis | Acceptable: ≥90% Achievable: ≥95% |
| DES-PS3 | To offer a timely appointment for DR screening to all known eligible people with diabetes, categorized under RDS | Proportion of eligible people offered an appointment for RDS occurring more than 6 weeks after their RDS recall due date | Acceptable: ≥95% Achievable: ≥98% |
| DES-PS4 | To offer a timely appointment for SLB screening to all people with diabetes on the SLB surveillance pathway | Proportion of eligible people offered an appointment for ongoing SLB surveillance occurring more than 6 weeks after their SLB recall due date | Acceptable: >60% Achievable: >85% |

**Table 12.1** Continued

| Standard | Objective | Description | Thresholds |
|---|---|---|---|
| DES-PS5 | To offer a timely appointment for digital surveillance to all people on the digital surveillance pathway | Proportion of due appointments for digital surveillance that have an offer of an appointment due to occur within a reasonable time of the follow-up period.<br>• *3 months*: ±1 week<br>• *4 and 5 months*: ±2 weeks<br>• *6 and 7 months*: ±3 weeks<br>• *8 and 9 months*: ±4 weeks<br>• *10 and 11 months*: ±5 weeks<br>• *12 months*: ±6 weeks | To be set |
| DES-PS6 | To maximize the number of pregnant women with diabetes seen in digital surveillance | Proportion of pregnant women with diabetes seen within 6 weeks of notification of their pregnancy to the screening provider | To be set |
| DES-PS7 | To maximize the number of invited people with diabetes receiving the test | Percentage of those offered RDS who attend an RDS event where images are captured | Acceptable: ≥75%<br>Achievable: ≥85% |
| DES-PS8 | To minimize the number of repeat non-attenders | Proportion of eligible people with diabetes who have not attended for screening in the previous 3 years | Acceptable: <80%<br>Achievable: <50% |
| DES-PS9 | To ensure digital images are of adequate quality | Proportion of eligible people with diabetes where a digital image has been obtained, but the final grading outcome is ungradable | Acceptable: between 2% and 4% |

*(continued)*

| Table 12.1 Continued | | | |
|---|---|---|---|
| Standard | Objective | Description | Thresholds |
| DES-PS10 | To ensure the person with diabetes, GP, and relevant health professionals are informed of test results | The proportion of eligible people with diabetes attending for diabetic eye screening, digital surveillance or SLB to whom results were issued within 3 weeks of the screening event | Acceptable: ≥70% within 3 weeks<br>Achievable: ≥95% within 3 weeks |
| DES-PS11 | To ensure timely referral of people with diabetes with positive screening results | Urgent referrals (R3A): time between routine digital screening event, or DS event, or SLB event, and issuing the referral to the HES | Acceptable: ≥95% within 2 weeks<br>Achievable: ≥98% within 2 weeks |
| | | Routine referrals (R2 or M1, including any referred as urgent): time between routine digital screening event or DS event or SLB event and issuing the referral to the HES | Acceptable: ≥90% within 3 weeks<br>Achievable: ≥95% within 3 weeks |
| DES-PS1 | To ensure timely consultation for people with diabetes who are screen positive | Urgent referrals (R3A): time between screening event and first attended consultation at HES or digital surveillance | Acceptable: ≥80% within 6 weeks |
| | | Routine referrals (R2 or M1, including any referrals as urgent): time between screening event and first attended consultation at HES or digital surveillance | Acceptable: ≥70% within 13 weeks<br>Achievable: ≥95% within 13 weeks |
| DES-PS13 | To ensure timely consultation for people with diabetes whose images are recorded as ungradable | Time between digital screening event and first attended consultation or SLB surveillance | Acceptable: ≥70% within 13 weeks<br>Achievable: ≥95% within 13 weeks |

RDS, routine digital surveillance; DR, diabetic retinopathy; SLB, slit lamp biomicroscopy; DS digital surveillance; HES, hospital eye service.

## 12.8 External quality assurance

It is important for a national screening programme that individual local programmes have external review to highlight issues causing difficulties and inconsistencies. All screening programmes in the UK have regular external quality assurance (EQA) with visits of senior trained screening personnel (i.e. peer review), occurring every 3 years. This peer-led multidisciplinary review process is overseen by the national screening quality assurance service (SQAS) team. The purpose of the visit is to:

- Review the quality of the screening programme.
- Identify risks.
- Identify areas of good/best practice.
- Mutual exchange of information/experience.
- Identify areas where improvements need to be made.
- Minimize harm and maximize benefits.
- Support the programme to achieve excellence.
- Ensure the visit has a fair and evidence-based approach.

In practice in the UK, most local DESPs are visited every three years by the external peer review process. This has been effective in achieving conformity, sustainability, and funding for programmes, as well as ensuring appropriate staffing and training.

FURTHER READING

Hamid A, Wharton HM, Mills A, Gibson JM, Clarke M, Dodson PM. (2016). Diagnosis of retinopathy in children younger than 12 years of age: implications for the diabetic eye screening guidelines in the UK. *Eye* **30**(7): 949–51.

Scanlon PH. (2017). The English National Screening Programme for diabetic retinopathy 2003–2016. *Acta Diabetol* **54**(6): 515–25.

Tye A, Wharton H, Wright A, Yang Y, Gibson J, Syed A, et al. (2015). Evaluating digital diabetic retinopathy screening in people aged 90 years and over. *Eye* **29**(11): 1442–5.

Wong TY, Sun J, Kawasaki R, Ruamviboonsuk P, Gupta N, Lansingh VC, et al. (2018). Guidelines on diabetic eye care: the International Council of Ophthalmology Recommendations for screening, follow-up, referral, and treatment based on resource settings. *Ophthalmology* **125**(10): 1608–22.

# CHAPTER 13

# Programme administration and fail-safe

Rebecca Smith

---

**KEY POINTS**

- Effective administration and fail-safe is essential to any screening programme.
- A clear structure needs to be in place, identifying roles and responsibilities.
- Procedures, policies, and regular audits need to be implemented throughout the programme, from identifying patients, to onward referral to the eye clinic.
- Fail-safe processes need to be in place as a back-up mechanism to ensure patient safety at all points in the pathway.
- The programme needs to have the capacity to produce performance reports on an *ad hoc* basis, to show how it is performing and to improve its service for its patients.

---

## 13.1 Key administration areas

The key roles in a screening programme include:

- Identifying the cohort.
- Inviting to screening.
- Reporting the outcome.
- Onward referrals to eye services.
- Fail-safe.
- Internal quality assurance/reporting.

## 13.2 Patient list for diabetic eye screening

Each diabetic eye screening programme (DESP) must be able to identify and invite all eligible subjects with diabetes at regular intervals. It is important to try and screen subjects within 3 months of their date of diabetes diagnosis. In the NHS Diabetic Eye Screening Programme (NHSDESP), an eligible subject or patient is classed as a 'Person diagnosed with diabetes mellitus (excluding gestational diabetes) aged 12 or over who have light perception or better in at least one eye'. To ensure that all of your population is identified, there should be a single collated list

(SCL) of patients who are eligible for screening within your programme boundary. This should be regularly compared with primary care (GP) diabetes databases, and updated to ensure all patients are on the SCL and their demographic details are correct. This allows for invitations for screening and results to be correctly sent. The data required for each of these patients are:

- NHS number (patient identification number).
- Full name.
- Date of birth.
- Address.
- Primary care practice details.

Additional information that would prove to be useful is ethnicity, gender, and preferred language for communication.

As the prevalence of diabetes is increasing, this list will increase and patients' details will change. Some patients may change address or primary-care clinician, and some will die. In the UK, all diabetic patients should be identified to the programme and practitioners within a particular primary-care practice should not refer patients to different programmes. This is especially important on programme borders, as it is vital to ensure conformity and, hence, patient safety. Patients can ask to be seen in another programme, but policies need to be in place to fail-safe these patients and to invite them back if they do not attend for screening elsewhere. In the UK, the DESP suggests that a single comprehensive list and a single call/recall centre would be most effective.

It is important to work closely with primary care to create, validate, and maintain on at least a quarterly basis this register of eligible patients. The programme has specific software packages to help with extraction of the eligible patients from GP (primary care) practices. One example is the software GP2DRS, which is an extraction tool that obtains all the eligible patients from primary-care systems and supplies the demographic information to the relevant screening programme on a monthly basis. There needs to be close collaboration with the primary-care physicians while setting up electronic extractions, in order to ensure that they code their patients correctly and study any anomalies. One example is the coding of diabetes in remission. It is recommended that after any definitive diagnosis of diabetes, the subject is offered lifelong screening, even if their diabetes resolves and they are no longer classed as being diabetic (except in steroid-induced cases). If the subject is classed as 'diabetes resolved' on the primary-care system, their details will not be sent to the screening programme via GP2DRS, but if they are classed as 'diabetes in remission', then they will come across in the patient extract. The primary-care physician also needs to be aware of obtaining patient consent when coding, to ensure that subjects who do not consent for screening do not have their information automatically passed to the screening programme, thereby giving rise to an information governance breach. It is the primary-care physician's responsibility to have the initial conversation with the diabetic subject and change the consent code if necessary.

Primary care should not be solely relied upon; it is worth establishing links with departments such as antenatal and paediatrics. These teams may be aware of subjects who are diabetic before primary care is. This is especially important with the antenatal patient to ensure that screening during pregnancy occurs in the first trimester.

In England, there is a national database of patient demographic data. It is a good tool to access as it provides instant access to information, for example, when you have the invite address wrong and, therefore, need to establish the correct address. It also aids in establishing where subjects have moved to, not only within your boundary, but elsewhere in the country, so recent screening results can be forwarded on to that programme for continued patient care. With a good IT infrastructure (see Chapter 14, 'Models of screening and information technology') in a screening programme, comparisons of the screening database can be made with this national demographic database and discrepancies can be highlighted. This is specifically useful to pick up patients who have recently died, so that inappropriate screening invitations are not sent out, which may cause distress to relatives.

It is very beneficial to keep the primary-care practice informed of their diabetic subjects on the SCL, their current screening state, and any recent results. Reports on their individual practice uptake, with comparisons with other local practices can help build good relationships and an awareness of screening.

## 13.3 Eligible patient categories

Not all patients 'eligible' for screening on the SCL should be sent an invitation for screening. Eligible patients are entitled to an offer of screening, but not all are deemed appropriate for screening. The eligible cohort can be separated into three categories as described by the NHSDESP (see Table 13.1).

Both the suspended and excluded subjects will not have annual invitations for screening, although they need to be audited on a regular basis to ensure that they are offered screening when/if necessary. All suspended patients in the eye clinics should have their status monitored at least once every 12 months to confirm that they are still in the care of ophthalmology and are having retinopathy checked for. If this cannot be established then, for safety, the patient should be offered screening in one of the programme's clinics.

A small number of subjects who are eligible for screening will not want to be part of the screening programme. If a diabetic subject has decided to opt out, it is very important that they have been given all of the necessary information for this to be an informed choice. In the UK programme, it is mandated that if the subject still wishes to opt out, then written confirmation should be gained stating how long they wish to opt out for, and this should be attached to the patient record and the primary-care practice informed. This is an important audit trail.

**Table 13.1** The three eligible patient categories

| | |
|---|---|
| (a) Invited for screening patients | Should receive annual invitations to attend for screening |
| (b) Suspended patients | Subjects are not invited, but are under separate assessment for DR:<br>*Eye clinic*: seen by a medical retinal specialist and the clinician has taken responsibility for their care<br>*Digital surveillance (DS)*: digital images are taken by the screening programme on a regular basis, e.g. every 6 months and compared with previous images to review disease progression<br>*Slit lamp*: for patients not assessable by RDS these subjects can be assessed in the programme slit-lamp clinics. They can remain on annual review until they are either assessable and can go back to routine screening, or they develop referable DR, at which point they need to be referred to the eye clinic for their care |
| (c) Excluded patients | Subjects are not invited and do not have their retinae checked for DR. This could either have been the choice of the subject and they have opted out, and confirmed this in writing; or it could be subjects who would *not* benefit from regular review using slit lamp or would *not* benefit from treatment if it was required |

No diabetic subject should be opted out permanently and they should be offered an invitation for screening after a maximum of 3 years. It should be made clear that they can return to the screening programme at any point.

All other excluded patients need to have written confirmation from either their primary-care physician or ophthalmologist that they are not suitable for screening. This should be audited annually and primary care informed of their excluded patients, in case they now need to be reinstated into the screening programme.

Reasons for exclusion are discussed in Table 13.2.

Patients who are registered as partially sighted or blind should not be automatically excluded from screening. Detecting and treating diabetic retinopathy (DR) may retain some precious sight. Only patients who have no perception of light in both eyes, which is irreversible, should not be invited for screening, as they are classed as ineligible.

Diabetic patients who have their DR checked in private health care should also be offered screening and asked to opt out if they wish. Diabetic subjects who reside in care homes, mental health institutions, or prisons within a programme's catchment area should also be invited for screening. They should only be excluded from screening for reasons stated above, even if they are not registered with a local primary-care practice.

**Table 13.2** Reasons for exclusion

| | |
|---|---|
| Physical or mental disability | A subject having either a physical or mental disability does not automatically exclude them from being screened and the programme should make every effort possible to screen a subject. Hospital transport may be necessary to bring a subject to their appointment who would otherwise have been classed as housebound |
| Terminal illness | A person with diabetes who is terminally ill should continue being screened for as long as they are capable and happy to do so. If treatment is possible, retaining sight could increase the quality of life for terminally ill patients. Their GP can make a decision to exclude the patient from screening if they feel that it is in the patient's best interest |

## 13.4 Call and recall

It is important to have a central call/recall system using dedicated screening software that is automatic, and can move the subjects along their pathway without intervention or with minimal manual intervention. Without this, a large amount of extra work is generated and may result in delays in patient care. The software should be able to automatically invite patients for screening at the correct time, and generate patient results and referrals letters to ophthalmology, and primary-care notifications. Correspondence can be posted or emailed to the relevant parties. It is recommended when printing letters that audits are kept of the number of letters generated compared with the number posted. Outsourcing to large printing companies can help save time and money. Emailing results to primary-care practices is beneficial if there are IT solutions in place to obtain the screening result and input it directly into their practice systems.

It is good practice to have one patient-dedicated phone line that takes you directly to the administration team who has direct access to the screening software.

## 13.5 Onward referrals

It is vital that there is good administration in place to ensure that any subjects referred to either a surveillance clinic or to the hospital eye service at grading have their appointments made. Checks need to be in place to ensure that all referrals are known about and if referring to local hospital eye clinics then good links with these teams need to be established. In most cases, the screening programme will send the referral to the eye clinic and it is then the eye clinic's responsibility to book the appointment. Getting confirmation that they have received the referral is important and makes up part of an audit trail. It is at this point that the eye clinic then takes over the care of the subject for DR until they are discharged. Once attending the eye clinic, patients are classed as 'suspended' from screening and, as mentioned previously, require regular auditing. It is important to track all referrals made to ensure that appointments have been made and that they are within the correct timescales. Evidence from audits is vital when highlighting any issues.

## 13.6 Fail-safe

Fail-safe is a back-up mechanism to ensure that if something goes wrong in the screening pathway, processes are in place to identify what has gone wrong, and action follows to ensure safe outcomes.

Fail-safe should happen along the whole screening pathway and it is everyone's responsibility. The main fail-safe areas where patients can fall through gaps and get lost are:

- Identifying and registering all eligible diabetic patients with correct demographic data.
- Sending all invitations and results letters, ensuring the number of letters generated matches the number printed.
- Attaching photographs to the correct patient record. Ensuring all screening retinal images are graded.
- Actioning all referrals to surveillance and the hospital eye clinics.
- Following up all suspended and excluded subjects, ensuring they are offered screening as and when necessary.

## 13.7 Incidents

All incidents identified in the screening programme should be reported, investigated, and acted upon. Action plans should be implemented to mitigate harm and prevent the incident happening again. Lessons can then be identified for wider dissemination. Incidents can be found by completing the audits. Examples include identifying subjects registered as sight-impaired and review if the screening programme fails the patient at any point in the pathway, e.g. late registration, or an audit of those identified with a new diagnosis of proliferative retinopathy to assess that they receive appropriate timely treatment.

## 13.8 Reporting

Reporting is a key administrative function and is used to identify:

- Data quality.
- Activity, e.g. number of new subjects registered, screening uptake.
- Timeliness of inviting and retinal image grading of subjects.

- Referral issues, e.g. highlighting problems with ophthalmology clinics and services.
- Subjects with delays in specific actions, e.g. patients suspended with no retinopathy grade for over a year.
- Trends or patterns that may need investigation, e.g. high exclusion rate compared with other screening programmes, or low uptake in specific areas. This may need addressing with plans implemented to improve uptake.
- Comparison of data on a national basis, e.g. effectiveness, trends, prevalence of DR, and performance against national standards compared with others.

A programme performance report is recommended to be made on a quarterly basis and compared with previous reports. It should help identify strengths and weaknesses of the programme. This enables review of all aspects and helps to identify areas that can be targeted where improvements are needed. The *standards* that are set for the NHSDESP are outlined in Table 12.1.

## 13.9  Summary

Effective administration and fail-safe is key to a successful screening programme, so that the correct subjects get an invitation, obtain an accurate quality assured screen, and receive timely results and treatment where necessary. The NHSDESP gives guidance on who should be offered screening and who should be excluded. There are many parts of the subject screening pathway in which patients can 'fall through gaps', emphasizing the importance of fail-safe, checking to identify these and prevent reoccurrence. Administration and fail-safe costs money, and this may cause problems for screening programmes in the short term, but in the longer term is of benefit in ensuring that all eligible subjects are invited or referred for treatment in a timely manner, thereby protecting vision and preventing blindness.

FURTHER READING

Gov.UK. (2013). Diabetic eye screening programme: failsafe procedures. https://www.gov.uk/government/publications/diabetic-eye-screening-programme-failsafe-procedures (accessed 20 August 2019).

Gov.UK. (2013). NHS diabetic eye screening (DES) programme. https://www.gov.uk/topic/population-screening-programmes/diabetic-eye (accessed 20 August 2019).

# CHAPTER 14

# Models of screening and information technology

Andrew Mills

---

**KEY POINTS**

- A screening service needs centralized storage, and a server computer to receive data from and send data to users.
- The user needs one local computer to collect or display patient information.
- All connections must be secure and meet current local data protection laws.
- The model of screening determines how best to transfer patient data between server and end users.
- Flexibility is key and may require a mixed approach to offer the greatest reach for screening.

---

## 14.1 Introduction

Ten years after the first edition, computing continues to evolve. Operating systems have moved on, and more of us are connected to the Internet to the point where 'broadband' is now a universal term and deemed to be a key service along with electricity to the home. Technology shrinks with fast, battery-powered devices (tablets and smart phones) are permanently connected via mobile data, and changes how we understand and what we do with the technology. Technology is now about convenience and communication, be it social media networks or tracking a parcel to your door, the computer behind the scene has been lost under the glossy screens of the latest must-have device.

This has affected screening, too. Remote computers can now be easily connected to the screening centre with a small mobile data dongle, and text messages to remind a patient about their upcoming appointment are commonplace. Behind the scenes, a well-developed, co-ordinated infrastructure residing in the background is as essential as ever. This infrastructure comes in the form of two key components:

- *'The Model'*: how data are collected and used.
- *The information technology (IT)*: required for shuffling data round the various components of the model.

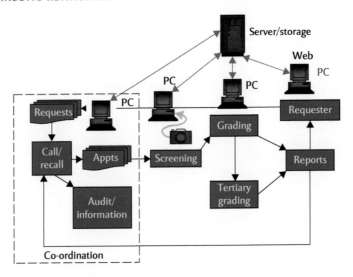

Figure 14.1 A typical workflow pattern showing data flow round the screening model. A hardware layer applied to this indicates how the data flow back and forth from the server and PCs.

Appts, appointments.

Reproduced courtesy of Professor Paul M. Dodson and The Heart of England Retinal Screening Centre.

Both are closely interrelated, but compromises between IT and screening programme needs have changed; better connectivity keeps remote stations in contact, and screening has evolved with new pathways to manage. The balance between efficacy and cost of provision of the scheme remains an issue. Urban and rural screening programmes share the typical workflow pattern shown in Figure 14.1, and both have unique variations that mean it is neither appropriate nor practical to enforce one model or one IT infrastructure onto a programme.

## 14.2 Information technology and screening

IT should sit in the background, quietly doing its job, relieving the user of repetitive chores and multiple data entry, not interfering with the screening process. The holy grail of any IT infrastructure is to have to enter the correct data *only once*, and with the advances in software design and computer power, all the tools we need for this are available today—it is certainly possible to have a seamless flow of data round the entire UK NHS entity, although lack of understanding, funding, interested parties protecting their ground, and the inevitable red-tape, means that this goal often has remained elusive. For the screening programme, however, we have moved forward. Primary-care systems now communicate data to the system; as do ophthalmology systems, so it is possible to automate some of the chores of data entry for new patients and updating details.

Screening programmes accumulate data centrally to ensure the needs of the patients are met, and for the programme to co-ordinate and monitor activity. This central repository is a computer, known as a *server*, connected to a large storage repository to hold the images, and the database that will be used to manage the dataset that is needed to identify each patient, image, and grade held on the system. Queries are asked of the data in the database, which allows screening programme administrators to send out appointments, results, and to audit the processes involved. Out in the community *client* computers (simple PCs) are used to collect and receive data from the server. Between the two lies a connection medium, which depends on the model of the screening programme.

## 14.3 Screening models

Common to all programme designs is a call/recall service, where the central service can recall patients when they are due for screening by means of an invitation letter. This invitation may use appointment booking systems, where patients ring and book appointments (*open booking*), or a system where appointments are sent to patients with the invitation (*closed booking*).

Open booking allows a subject the flexibility to choose a time and place, or indeed, perhaps to just drop in to a screening location. This does come at the cost of advance planning and some monitoring of rates of non-attendance. Both methodologies have disadvantages; open booking suffers from people not bothering to respond, while closed booking suffers from non-attenders and wasted appointment slots. Flexibility is key here—being able to offer both types in the same programme has merit; strangely, patients who would not respond to open invites will sometimes attend a prebooked appointment, particularly if it is in a 'medical' (e.g. hospital or equivalent facility) location.

Two screening models represent the different approaches to implementing retinal screening. One is an indirect model, where remote screeners take images, collected locally from the client and send in the data later. The other is a directly connected model, where data are transferred back and forth to the server from the client immediately (in IT parlance this is known as real-time). Between these two models are combinations that may suit the retinal screening programme being developed. No one model is a perfect solution, and several compromises may be needed along the way. In rural areas, a screener with a van containing the camera and computer driving to a point to provide retinal screening for the day can be far more cost-effective than providing several fixed camera locations with network connections and staff for relatively low levels of population density. In urban areas, where population density is high, fixed locations and direct connection will provide better access to the screening programme.

## 14.4 Model 1: remote data collection

In this model a screener/grader travels to locations for a screening session in a suitably equipped van with camera and computer to reach remote communities in locales that demand a different approach to providing a retinal screening programme. Targeting specific locales on a regular basis can serve the needs of a population far more effectively than asking service users to visit a screening centre many miles away. Here, the operator takes images, collects them on the local PC, and either grades locally or later, having uploaded the images back at the screening centre. However, this method brings about a challenge to data integrity and transfer—how to make sure the right data are in the right place at the right time.

The solution is a secure messaging structure built into the software governing transfer of data between client and server. The local PC in the van is then treated as a miniature screening programme, and the one machine is its own server, image store, database, and client application. Data can then be transferred from the PC when the van returns to its home location or when it reaches a suitable connection to gain access to the screening network. If enough security can be ensured, by utilizing virtual private networks (VPNs—where a private network is created over a public network and appears to the user as a direct connection to the private network), A cloud or mobile data connection could be also utilized to transfer data when the van is parked. Indeed, many Internet service providers can now offer a guaranteed direct secure data connection back to the server, and if there was sufficient mobile phone signal in an area, the potential is there to have a secure direct connection back to base operating in real-time. This has to be tempered with the fact that, by moving round, the van may well move to locations with poor signals, preventing a connection.

Mobile locations fit well with a closed appointment system, where the potential attendance is known in advance. The disadvantage is that a subject failing to attend wastes those precious booking slots and, thus, there is less efficient use of the mobile facility; adding drop-in facilities risks the possibility of over-crowding and potentially turning away patients. Indeed, patients turning up unannounced may have to be re-registered on the local system to be screened or turned away as the database will not contain a complete set of patient registrations, but simply the data required to screen the patients already booked.

## 14.5 Model 2: indirect remote locations

With much improved connectivity and the use of VPNs over the last 10 years, this option is now somewhat redundant. The halfway house between the mobile van and a direct connection, indirect remote locations are fixed locations in the community appointed to screen subjects for the screening programme (and possibly primary grade), but with no direct connection to base.

Again, the local PC is a miniature screening programme in its own right, with no direct link to base; it must contain all necessary data ahead of time communicating to the central server by a messaging system. It works best with closed appointments; the same caveats apply regarding non-attendance and drop-in sessions.

## 14.6 Model 3: directly connected locations

Here, the client PC is directly connected to the servers, through an approved secure connection. The PC may be located in a doctor's surgery or outreach clinic, or a specially connected optometrist's practice. The screening service may employ an optometrist in a practice for the purposes of screening with a suitable contract to cover information governance requirements. No messaging is required at this point and the information is never stored permanently on the local system. This model brings about some very different problems and some very important advantages for the screening programme. Notably, the appointment and subject data are pulled from the server in real-time with images and grading data uploaded to the main server the instant it is collected. Here, it is possible to ensure the ideal of only having to enter patient registration data once is viable as far as the screening programme is concerned. In addition, should there be an urgent need to review a patient by an ophthalmologist, the real-time nature of data transfer would allow this. Indeed, cross-pollination of ideas in this instance is much easier, as graders can easily bring patients up for review while on the telephone to their colleagues reviewing the same images for advice. This model lends itself well to more urban areas where population densities are much higher, with larger numbers of permanent screening locations open for longer hours, and up to 7 days a week with an open appointments system where subjects are invited by letter to attend for screening, rather than being sent an appointment. The location can also host informal drop-in sessions, whereby people simply walk in for screening. The difficulty with such locations, however, may be maintaining a high standard of information governance, as staff may no longer be under direct employment of the screening service. It is therefore essential to have protocols, training facilities, and quality-control checking in place if this route is chosen.

Of particular concern to retinal screening is the hard-to-reach groups—those patients in residential care homes, the housebound, or prison populations. These people are fixed populations, where it is possible to book appointments in advance and screen, at a location where direct connection to the server would probably not be possible. Here, coupling a mobile service with fixed directly connected locations allows coverage of the widest of the diabetic population.

## 14.7 Data transfer

Screening models must transfer data between the client PC and server. To do this, either the software must create a message set of all relevant patient data and 'post' it between the client and server, receiving more data in return; or communicate in real-time with the server along secure pathways. Both methods must be securely encrypted so that no one can read the data without the proper credentials.

A messaging solution can make use of any medium, from USB memory sticks, via optical storage, through to a VPN connection to the server, while the directly connected method must have a direct connection to the server using a network either via a secure network or over a public connection using a VPN connection to the server.

Each method has its advantages and disadvantages—optical media and USB memory sticks can be lost, corrupted, or damaged in transit; media must be encrypted and password protected in order to prevent information escaping in the event of a physical media loss. In their favour is that there is no need to be close to a network connection; this is useful in remote locations, too far away from a broadband connection.

The direct connection model relies heavily on permanent, stable, securely encrypted connections to the server, something not always guaranteed as anyone with experience of such a system will tell you. Any faults are guaranteed only to occur on the busiest afternoon!

## 14.8 Software and automation

Software programs are the tools we use on a computer to record, and co-ordinate the collection and processing of data. There are several commercial software systems available, specifically designed for DR screening. In setting up a new programme, either designing a screening software system in-house or purchasing one already available is of paramount importance to the success of screening. Experience in Africa, using early software of capture and grading only, led to the patient details and pathways being performed manually, with substantial staffing and the obvious inherent problems.

Automation of grading is topical at present, and is a clear way forward to aid a DR screening system. Several softwares have and are being developed to aid in the differentiation between no disease and disease (i.e. normal or abnormal), or actually producing a retinal grade. The former has been tested in the Scottish programme and has an appropriate sensitivity for detection of abnormal data. Automated grading systems are in the validation process for grading DR in retinal photographs and, indeed, also interpretation of optical coherence tomography (OCT) images. It is likely that automation and artificial intelligence will play a large part in digital retinal screening in the future, as being demonstrated in a number of recent publications. The use of the smartphone in combination with artificial intelligence looks promising, particularly in rural populations with limited access to IT.

## 14.9 Summary

A screening service needs infrastructure to operate, servers to store data, client machines to collect the data, secure data networks to transfer information safely, and dedicated personnel to drive the service. Lying on top of this is the service model, whether to use open or closed booking, fixed or mobile locations. No one method is king and, in most cases, there is much to be gained from mixing methods.

FURTHER READING

Fleming AD, Philip S, Goatman KA, Prescott GJ, Sharp PF, Olson JA. ( 2011). The evidence for automated grading in diabetic retinopathy screening. *Curr Diabetes Rev* 7(4): 246–52.

Gov.UK. (2014). UK National Screening Committee. Diabetic eye screening: programme overview. https://www.gov.uk/guidance/diabetic-eye-screening-programme-overview (accessed 20 August 2019).

Jesus DA, Barbosa Breda J, Van Keer K, Rocha Sousa A, Abegão Pinto L, Stalmans I. (2019). Quantitative automated circumpapillary microvascular density measurements: a new angioOCT-based methodology. *Eye (Lond)* 33(2): 320–6.

Kapetanakis VV, Rudnicka AR, Liew G, Owen CG, Lee A, Louw V, et al. (2015). A study of whether automated diabetic retinopathy image assessment could replace manual grading steps in the English National Screening Programme. *J Med Screen* 22(3): 112–18.

Rajalakshmi R, Subashini R, Anjana RM, Mohan V. (2018). Automated diabetic retinopathy detection in smartphone-based fundus photography using artificial intelligence. *Eye (Lond)* 32(6): 1138–44.

Ribeiro L, Oliveira CM, Neves C, Ramos JD, Ferreira H, Cunha-Vaz J. (2016). Screening for diabetic retinopathy in the central region of Portugal. Added value of automated 'disease/no disease' grading. *Ind J Opthalmol* 64(1): 26–32.

# CHAPTER 15

# Training and accreditation for retinal screening and grading

Karen Whitehouse

**KEY POINTS**

- In all national screening programmes, staff training and accreditation will be required for patient safety.
- This chapter sets out how the UK programme has evolved in this aspect.
- The current NHS Diabetic Eye Screening Programme (NHSDESP) training requirement for personnel undertaking screening, grading, and slit lamp will be explained, as well as the NVQ level 3 qualification: 'Health Screener: diabetic eye screening'.
- All grading staff should also participate in test and training retinal image sets, in order to confirm accuracy of grading.

## 15.1 Introduction

An expectation and requirement on any screening programme is that staff should be properly trained and accredited for their job. While screening programmes have been well established for other conditions, the basic principles of screening and training are common to the NHSDESP, but the training for the more specialist nature of the programme with digital image capture and grading has led to the development of new qualifications. Indeed, these have evolved from a diploma with City and Guilds in London to the current qualifications.

## 15.2 Accreditation of competence

A *Level 3 Health Screener Award* has been developed as an accreditation of the minimum level of competence required by *all* personnel involved in the preparation of the patient for screening, undertaking imaging, and assessing images for grading. This qualification supersedes the City and Guilds qualification.

The qualification confirms that the learner has been fully assessed against the standards set for the profession and has fulfilled the required criteria. Principally, it is designed to protect the patient, but also protects the worker and employer.

Ultimately, it is hoped it will encourage the recruitment and retention of staff.

By undertaking the mandatory units, the health screener has completed all units required to specialize in their role—the mandatory units are the same for all health screeners (abdominal aortic aneurysm, newborn hearing, and diabetic eye screening programmes [DESPs]).

## 15.3 NHS population screening: qualification for health screeners

The level 3 diploma for health screeners and graders is the required training programme for all new diabetic eye screeners who are not already a trained healthcare professional.

This qualification has been developed by a multidisciplinary reference group comprising of subject experts.

There are four awarding bodies:

- Futurequals.
- Innovate Awarding.
- National Open College Network.
- Pearson Qualifications.

There are awarding centres available to register the learner, who will supply learner material, assessor documents, quality assurance, certification submission, and support. The award is comprised of:

- 13 mandatory units;
- five role-specific units, plus safeguarding.

If the learner is only required to undertake specific parts of the qualification, they will be awarded certificates to show that they are competent in that speciality.

The mandatory units are:

1. Engage in personal development in health, social care, or children's and young people's settings.
2. Promote communication in health, social care, or children's and young people's settings.
3. Promote equality and inclusion in health, social care, or children's and young people's settings.
4. Promote and implement health and safety in health and social care.
5. Principles of safeguarding and protection in health and social care.
6. Promote person-centred approaches in health and social care.
7. The role of the health and social care worker.

8. Promote good practice in handling information in health and social care settings.

9. The principles of infection prevention and control.

10. Causes and spread of infection.

11. Cleaning, decontamination, and waste management.

12. Principles for implementing duty of care in health, social care, or children's and young people's settings.

13. Health screening principles.

The role-specific units are:

1. Anatomy, physiology, and pathology of the eye.

2. Understanding diabetes and diabetic retinopathy

3. Prepare for diabetic retinopathy screening.

4. Undertake diabetic retinopathy imaging.

5. Detect retinal disease and classify diabetic retinopathy.

6. Understand how to safeguard the well-being of children and young people.

A screener who does not grade would be required to complete:

- All mandatory units *plus*:
  - Anatomy, physiology, and pathology of the eye.
  - Understanding diabetes and diabetic retinopathy.
  - Prepare for diabetic retinopathy screening.
  - Undertake diabetic retinopathy imaging.
  - Understand how to safeguard the well-being of children and young people.

A grader who does not screen would be required to complete:

- All mandatory units *plus*:
  - Anatomy, physiology, and pathology of the eye.
  - Understanding diabetes and diabetic retinopathy.
  - Detect retinal disease and classify diabetic retinopathy.

A screener/grader would be required to complete the whole qualification.

Each unit has been assessed as requiring a specific number of hours to complete them, expressed as guided learning hours.

Optometrists are only required to complete:

- Health-screening Principles.
- Understanding Diabetes and diabetic retinopathy.

- Prepare for diabetic retinopathy screening.
- Undertake diabetic retinopathy imaging.
- Detect retinal disease and classify diabetic retinopathy—*if the role requires.*

Other candidates who have previous qualifications should contact the Awarding Centre for details, as certain units may be subject to the RPL process.

Additional units must be taken by candidates if their job role extends beyond their original qualification requirement.

Continuing competence is achieved through continuing professional development and is measured by performance indicators (internal and external quality assurance [QA]) in the national screening programmes, and appraisals.

Details of all approved rules of combination can be found via gov.uk and the link can be found in the further reading.

## 15.4 Training for slit lamp examiners

The NHSDESP slit lamp biomicroscopy (SLB) examiner training and accreditation framework has been produced to assist programmes with the training of staff to become slit lamp examiners.

An accredited slit lamp examiner in NHSDESP can be:

- An ophthalmologist, consultant, associate specialist, staff grade, or specialist registrar year III (or higher) with at least 1 year's experience of medical retina clinics, and an understanding and the ability to follow the NHSDESP grading criteria.

*Or:*

- A grader who:
  o has completed the full diploma for health screeners qualification; *or*
  o has completed the previous City and Guilds diploma in diabetic retinopathy (DR) screening and completed the units 3, 4, 5, 7, and 8;
  o is working within a local diabetic eye screening (DES) service as a grader, grading at least 1000 image sets per year;
  o is participating in the monthly test and training sets;
  o has completed the assessment/accreditation process.

*Or:*

- A qualified practicing optometrist registered with the General Optical Council (GOC):

- Optometrists registered with the GOC who are just undertaking SLB within NHSDESP need to complete the 'Detect retinopathy and classify diabetic retinopathy unit' of the diploma for health screeners.
- Optometrists who have completed unit 7 and 8 in the previous City and Guilds qualification are exempt from taking additional units if undertaking SLB only. If optometrists are undertaking full disease grading within the local DES service, they must also complete the appropriate units for the roles they have within the screening programme.
- The optometrist should be participating in the monthly test and training sets.
- They should have completed the assessment/accreditation process.

The framework units consist of:

- Level one/preliminary training: supervised SLB examination technique.
- Level one/preliminary assessment.
- Level two/supervised grading of DR and related disorders using SLB.
- Level two/final assessment.

Completion of this requires close partnership between screening programmes and Ophthalmology; an SLB assessor should be an ophthalmologist.

Screening programmes may opt for their own competence framework alongside their Ophthalmology Department, but the learner must be deemed proficient and safe to practice, and should be assessed regularly to ensure competence is maintained.

## 15.5 Test and training

Any grader who is registered on the local programme management software and grades regularly, is expected to comply with this guidance. This should include optometrists, medical staff, consultant ophthalmologists, and consultant diabetologists involved in DES.

Ten test sets of retinal images should be completed annually, but for graders it is good practice to complete a test each month to see how they are grading in comparison with national guidelines. It should not be the sole standard for graders, as they should be assessed alongside their 'live' grading standards, i.e. intergrader reports.

Test and training sets are supplied via the Gloucester Retinal Education Group. Graders with the highest sensitivity and specificity results are invited to be part of a Grader College, which meets to discuss test and training protocols, and who are also responsible for grading image sets before they are issued nationally.

Since 2012, all images/cases have been approved for use only after '3 of 3' agreement by members of the National Grading College.

An international test and training (iTAT) facility has been produced via the Grading College centre in Gloucester for graders outside of NHSDESP.

## 15.6 Training courses

The Birmingham Diabetic Eye Screening Programme provides training courses for national and international learners.

There are two main courses.

### 15.6.1 Introduction to diabetic retinopathy grading

This is a course designed to provide the learner with in-depth training on DR grading, with lectures on how to grade, other eye disease encountered in retinal screening, and quizzes to assess the candidate's progress throughout.

### 15.6.2 Advanced diabetic retinopathy grading

This is a clinical-biased course for graders, senior graders, and referral outcome graders, who wish to further their knowledge of DR grading.

## 15.7 British Association of Retinal Screening

Since 2001, the British Association of Retinal Screening (BARS) has been the UK's professional organization for those who provide retinal screening services for people with diabetes. BARS offers education, representation, and support to a wide range of professionals, and is free to join.

BARS is a not-for-profit organization, run by an elected council with varying specialties, who meet regularly and also manage the annual conference. All members are entitled to attend this event.

FURTHER READING

Birmingham, Solihull and Black Country Diabetic Eye Screening. Training courses overview. http://www.retinalscreening.co.uk/training/training-courses/ (accessed 21 August 2019).

British Association for Retinal Screening (BARS). (2017). https://www.eyescreening.org.uk (accessed 21 August 2019).

Gov.UK. (2017). Diabetic eye screening: slit lamp biomicroscopy training. https://www.gov.uk/government/publications/diabetic-eye-screening-slit-lamp-biomicroscopy-training (accessed 21 August 2019).

Gov.UK. (2017). Diabetic eye screening: test and training participation. https://www.gov.uk/government/publications/diabetic-eye-screening-test-and-training-participation (accessed 21 August 2019).

Gov.UK. (2017). NHS population screening: diploma for health screeners. https://www.gov.uk/guidance/nhs-population-screening-diploma-for-health-screeners (accessed 21 August 2019).

https://www.gov.uk/government/publications/des-diploma-for-health-screeners-rules-of-combination

# CHAPTER 16

# Medical management of diabetic retinopathy

Paul M. Dodson

**KEY POINTS**

- Medical management is focused on the proven benefit of tight glucose and blood pressure (BP) control.
- Standard management includes multiple cardiovascular risk factor management with angiotensin receptor blockade, statin, and fibrate treatment.
- Targets to achieve include HbA1C <7% (53 mmol/mol), BP <140/80, and serum cholesterol <4 mmol/L.
- A number of large recent trials have specifically demonstrated the beneficial effects on diabetic retinopathy (DR) of angiotensin receptor blockade (the DIRECT study) and fenofibrate (the Fenofibrate Intervention and Event Lowering in Diabetes [FIELD] and Action to Control Cardiovascular Risk in Diabetes [ACCORD]-Eye studies).

## 16.1 Clinical need

One of the most feared complications of diabetes is blindness and loss of vision. There has, therefore, been extensive clinical and laboratory research to target this complication, and progress has been made. Although the retinal leakage may be influenced by medical treatment, once capillary closure and ischaemia is extensive then medical therapies will have little impact. This is also the case when there is significant macula ischaemia and visual loss, such that retinal laser treatment is contraindicated, and no effective medical therapy is known. Ischaemic maculopathy, therefore, remains a common cause of visual loss in diabetic subjects until the advent of intra-vitreal anti-vascular endothelial growth factor (VEGF) treatment. The basic management of Types 1 and 2 diabetes are outlined in Chapter 1, 'What is diabetes?'.

## 16.2 Conventional risk factor modification

### 16.2.1 Glycaemia and blood pressure

To achieve optimal glycaemic control requires the input of a multidisciplinary team to provide education and motivation for the diabetic patient. This will include general practitioners (GPs) in close collaboration with other members of the health-care team, including the practice and diabetes specialist nurses, dietitian, chiropodist, and psychologist (where appropriate), as well as the diabetes specialist care team.

The United Kingdom Prospective Diabetes Study (UKPDS), and the Diabetes Control and Complications Trial (DCCT) have confirmed, beyond question, the benefit of improving glycaemic control in patients with both Types 1 and 2 diabetes. Both these studies achieved a target glycated haemoglobin of around 7% (a measure of average glucose control over a 6–8-week period) with major reductions in microvascular complications. Any reduction in glycated haemoglobin was of benefit and there was no threshold effect.

The DCCT trial in patients with Type 1 diabetes demonstrated that intensive insulin treatment achieving a 2% difference in glycosylated haemoglobin resulted in a 76% reduction of developing new retinopathy. Similarly, in the UKPDS in Type 2, diabetes every 1% reduction in glycosylated haemoglobin translated into a 37% reduction of microvascular complications (see Figure 16.1). The ocular microvascular endpoints reduced progression of DR, laser requirement, and cataract formation.

Importantly, the idea of metabolic memory or legacy effect of good glycaemic control on retinopathy has been demonstrated by both the DCCT and UKPDS studies. In the DCCT/Epidemiology of Diabetes Interventions and Complications (EDIC) study after 10 years follow-up, where the glycated haemoglobin levels had converged completely, the former intensive treatment group still had 24% reduction in progression of retinopathy and 59% reduction in proliferative retinopathy, but the risk reductions at 10 years were attenuated compared with the first 4 years of follow-up. In the UKPDS despite glycated haemoglobin differences being lost after the first year in the sulphonyl

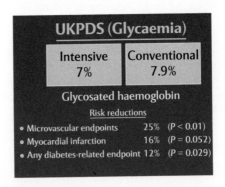

Figure 16.1 Summary of the UKPDS trial—blood glucose control.
Reproduced courtesy of Professor Paul M. Dodson and The Heart of England Retinal Screening Centre.

urea–insulin treatment group, relative reductions in risk persisted at 10 years for any diabetes-related endpoint (9%, $P = 0.04$) and for microvascular disease (24%, $P = 0.001$).

There are no diabetic drugs with specific efficacy in altering DR except by altering glucose control. However, owing to the possible 2.6-fold increase in macular oedema associated with the use of thiazolidinediones (e.g. pioglitazone), but not with other anti-diabetic drugs, current advice is to withdraw pioglitazone when macular oedema has developed.

## 16.3 Recommendations for management of glycaemia

A personalized HbA1C target should be set, usually between 48 and 58 mmol/mol (6.5–7.5%). No threshold level of glycaemia has been shown in any of the larger studies of retinopathy.

Less strict targets should be set (NICE quality standards, June 2011) in patients with established cardiovascular disease and in older subjects.

Patients should receive an on-going review of treatment to minimize hypoglycaemia.

Pioglitazone should be avoided in the presence of macular oedema.

### 16.3.1 Blood pressure control

Tight control of BP is also crucial as has been demonstrated in many large treatment trials. The UKPDS specifically studied microvascular endpoints, showing a 37% reduction in Type 2 diabetic patients achieving a systolic BP of 144 mmHg at 7 years follow-up (see Figure 16.2), and a 34% reduction in the proportion of patients with deterioration of retinopathy severity. The risk of microvascular

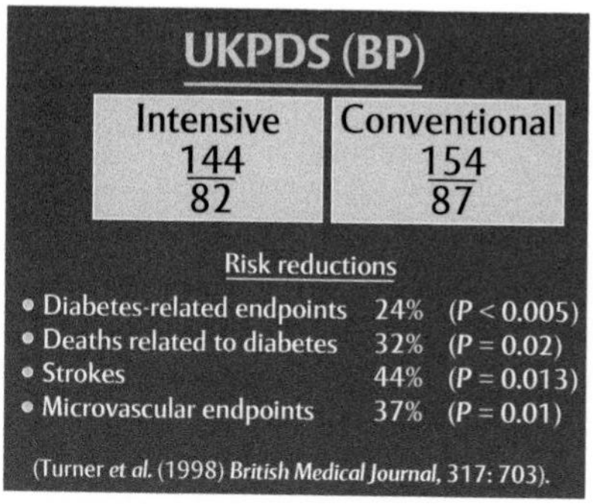

**UKPDS (BP)**

| Intensive | Conventional |
|:---:|:---:|
| 144 | 154 |
| 82 | 87 |

Risk reductions
- Diabetes-related endpoints   24%   ($P < 0.005$)
- Deaths related to diabetes   32%   ($P = 0.02$)
- Strokes   44%   ($P = 0.013$)
- Microvascular endpoints   37%   ($P = 0.01$)

(Turner et al. (1998) *British Medical Journal*, 317: 703).

Figure 16.2 **Summary of the UKPDS BP lowering study.**
Reproduced courtesy of Professor Paul M. Dodson and The Heart of England Retinal Screening Centre.

complications was reduced by 11% per 10 mmHg decrease in systolic BP. No legacy effect was demonstrated so BP control should be maintained to be effective.

### 16.3.2 Guidelines for hypertension in diabetes

- Intensify therapy aiming for systolic BP ≤130 mmHg in those with established retinopathy and/or nephropathy (level A).
- Encourage regular monitoring of BP in a health-care setting and at home if possible.
- Recognize that lower pressures may be beneficial overall, but evidence is lacking for retinopathy (level B).
- Recognize that specific therapies blocking the renin–angiotensin system (RAS) may have additional benefits, particularly for mild retinopathy, but should be discontinued during pregnancy (level B).

Almost all people with diabetes will require a combination of BP lowering drugs to achieve recommended targets, but some will require three or more. This combination is likely to include an angiotensin-converting enzyme (ACE) or angiotensin receptor blocker (ARB) in view of their specific effects described below.

## 16.4 Angiotensin receptor blockade

The ARBs are gaining more trial evidence of benefit, particularly in nephropathy and are now being widely used. Evidence for renin–angiotensin system blockade is strongest for nephroprotection (kidney disease). A role for angiotensin has been suggested in in vitro experiments in retinal angiogenesis and tested in people with diabetes. The EURODIAB Controlled Trial of Lisinopril in Insulin-Dependent Diabetes (EUCLID) study suggested the potential of specific treatment of ACE inhibition (lisinopril) to DR with 45% reduction of progression, but the study conclusion was confounded by better glucose control in the lisinopril group compared with control.

A large randomized landmark trial of an ARB (candesartan in the DIabetic Retinopathy Candesartan Trial (DIRECT) study) demonstrated—in 5231 diabetic patients after 5 years of candersartan treatment in Type 1 diabetes—a reduction in the incidence of retinopathy by two or more steps (Early Treatment Diabetic Retinopathy Study [EDTRS] scale) in severity by 18%, but no effect on progression of established retinopathy. In contrast, in Type 2 diabetes, 5 years of candersartan treatment resulted in a 34% regression of retinopathy. Importantly, an overall significant change towards less severe retinopathy was noted in both Type 1 and Type 2 diabetes.

While it is clear that the effects of increasing BP and glycaemic control are risk factors for microvascular disease, importantly these are *additive* as shown in the analysis from the UKPDS study and illustrated in Figure 16.3.

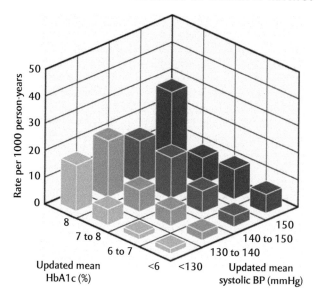

Figure 16.3 The additive risk factors for worsening glycaemic control as measured by glycated haemoglobin and systolic BP in the UKPDS.

Adapted with permission from Stratton IM, Cull CA, Adler AI, Matthews DR, Neil HAW, Holman RR. (2006). Additive effects of glycaemia and blood pressure exposure on risk of complications in type 2 diabetes: a prospective observational study (UKPDS 75), *Diabetologia*, 49(8): 1761–9. © 2006, Springer-Verlag. https://doi.org/10.1007/s00125-006-0297-1.

## 16.4.1 Lipid lowering therapy

Statin therapy has been proven to reduce cardiovascular disease in diabetic patients in both primary and secondary prevention, such that most Type 2 diabetic patients should be on this group of drugs, unless there is a contraindication or drug intolerance. Fibrate agents are widely used for treatment of predominantly increased triglyceride levels, commonly in association with low levels of high density lipoprotein (HDL) cholesterol, but have less effect on cardiovascular disease in Type 2 diabetes than statins.

More recently, data have confirmed that increasing total cholesterol and low density lipoprotein (LDL) levels, as well as increasing fasting serum triglycerides, is associated with a greater risk of developing maculopathy and macular oedema (see Chapter 4, 'Diabetes and the eye').

The Collaborative Atorvastatin Diabetes Study (CARDS) assessed the effectiveness of atorvastatin 10 mg daily versus placebo for primary prevention of cardiovascular events in patients with Type 2 diabetes (Colhoun et al., 2004). Over 4 years, the results from CARDS demonstrated a trend to reduction of laser therapy undertaken in the atorvastatin arm by 21%, which did not reach statistical significance and there was no influence on DR progression. Thus, the influence of statins on DR remains debatable, but if there is an effect, it is likely to be small.

The FIELD study, a large randomized trial designed to study the effects of the fibrate agent fenofibrate 200 mg/day compared with placebo, included the evaluation of microvascular endpoints. There was a highly significant 30% reduction in laser eye treatment in diabetic patients previously treated with fenofibrate. First laser treatment for macular oedema was reduced by 31% and for proliferative retinopathy by 30%. While there was no effect on primary prevention, those patients with pre-existing retinopathy at entry to the trial benefited most, i.e. in secondary prevention.

The ACCORD-Eye study has demonstrated that fenofibrate, in combination with a statin, resulted in a 40% reduction in odds of retinopathy progressing over 4 years compared with statin alone, such that fenofibrate should be considered for patients with pre-proliferative DR and/or diabetic maculopathy. These treatment benefits were not related to lipid levels or lowering thereof.

## 16.5 Aspirin

Diabetic patients with DR can take aspirin therapy, not because of a beneficial effect on DR, but due to the benefit of this agent, comprising a reduction in cardiovascular disease events in this cohort of patients, which was demonstrated some years ago in the EDTRS study of laser treatment. Aspirin may be associated with increased haemorrhage, which could be deleterious to DR, particularly with fragile new vessel formation in proliferative retinopathy. However, trials of this potential effect have not shown any deleterious effect on retinal and vitreous haemorrhage.

### 16.5.1 Obstructive sleep apnoea

Obstructive sleep apnoea (OSA) has recently been identified as a risk factor for diabetic complications, including retinopathy. OSA belongs to a spectrum of breathing disorders during sleep that ranges from simple snoring to complete cessation of breathing. OSA is associated with several pathophysiological deficits found in DR. Hence, it is plausible that OSA could play a role in the pathogenesis of sight-threatening diabetic retinopathy (STDR).

Several studies have shown that OSA is associated with STDR in patients with Type 2 diabetes and is an independent predictor for the progression to pre-proliferative/proliferative DR. Continuous positive airway pressure treatment has been associated with reduction in pre-proliferative/proliferative DR. The missing part of this story is that interventional studies are needed to assess the impact of OSA treatment on STDR.

## 16.6 Multi-factorial interventions

The clinical trial evidence for treatment benefit for diabetic microvascular disease is largely based on single risk factor interventions. However, the Steno-2 study has provided some data on the benefits of a multi-factorial intervention programme. Type 2 diabetes patients were randomly allocated to an intensive treatment programme of drugs targeting glycaemia, lowering BP, and lipid lowering, in addition to specific treatment with ACE inhibition, statins, and aspirin. Over a 7.8-year period, there was a large benefit in reduction of cardiovascular disease endpoints by 53%, diabetic nephropathy by 61%, and DR progression by 58%. However, there was still progression of DR in 25% of patients, despite intensive treatment; hence, the concept of residual risk.

The management guidelines used in the Steno-2 study make up the current therapeutic approach advised for patients with diabetes. This approach does require considerable poly-pharmacy and multiple drugs, but more combinations of commonly used drugs are becoming available.

## 16.6.1 Ophthalmology and management of diabetes

In the UK, most patients have their diabetes care in a primary medical or nursing setting, so the ophthalmologist often provides the first specialist consultation. Ophthalmologists have an important role in the management of diabetic patients, since retinopathy heralds a significant stage of diabetes with evidence of microangiopathy.

- Systems can be set up to provide enhanced care for diabetic patients in eye clinics. For example, in addition to visual acuity and ocular assessments, BP measurements, and survey of other diabetes-related care and outcomes, can be performed routinely.

- The ophthalmologists can take the opportunity to ensure appropriate care and medical targets are being pursued. A number of simple, key questions (Box 16.1) may help determine whether patients have been lost to regular supervision or whether more specialized diabetes interventions are required.

---

**Box 16.1** Medical questions for patients with diabetic retinopathy

1. Who helps you to look after your diabetes? General practitioner, specialist diabetes nurse in community/GP surgery, in hospital or diabetes centre, or diabetes specialist.

2. When is your next appointment?

3. What is your long-range diabetes test result? Glycated haemoglobin (HbA1C) or fructosamine, when was the last test done?

3. What is your usual blood pressure? How often it is checked? Measured at home, measured in surgery or clinic.

4. Do you know what your blood cholesterol level is?

5. What is your current treatment?

---

- The same principles also apply to on-going follow-up of patients in the hospital eye service (HES), especially if laser therapy or intra-vitreal injection therapy is being considered.

## 16.7 New potential therapies for diabetic retinopathy

There are five main chemical pathways implicated in the pathogenesis of diabetic microvascular complications:

- Increased polyol pathway flux.
- Increased advanced glycation endproduct (AGE) formation.
- Activation of the protein kinase C (PKC) isoforms.
- Increased hexosamine pathway flux.
- Increased angiogenic growth factors, e.g. VEGF, growth hormone, and angiotensins.

Specific inhibitors of each of these pathways have been tested as shown in Figure 16.4, which combines the vascular changes, as well as the metabolic pathways leading to the retinal leakage and ischaemia fundamental to development of DR.

The first therapeutic approach tested in large clinical trials was of aldose reductase inhibitors. This group of drugs blocks the accumulation of excess intracellular sorbitol derived in the presence of hyperglycaemia. The retinal studies demonstrated a weak effect on microaneurysm formation, but had an unfavourable side effect profile, so are not in clinical use, but other related AGE inhibitors may eventually find a place in the management of diabetes. The second pathway is the increased free radical formation and oxidative stress in diabetic subjects, which have a plausible mechanism of injury. However, clinical trials of anti-oxidants, and vitamins C or E, have been largely disappointing.

More recent emphasis has been placed on human trials of DR focusing on newer agents that showed promising early results. These have included the PKC inhibitors (ruboxistaurin), and growth factor inhibition (growth hormone and insulin-like growth factor [IGF]-1) modulation with somastatin LAR and pegvisomant. In large randomized trials of patients with DR these agents have shown no conclusive evidence of benefit.

However, there has been a major advance with the advent of the use of intra-vitreal therapies, which are licensed for use in treatment of age-related macula degeneration and diabetic macular oedema. These are outlined in Chapter 20, 'New treatment strategies for diabetic eye disease', but will be reserved for patients with more advanced retinopathy, rather than in the early development of DR.

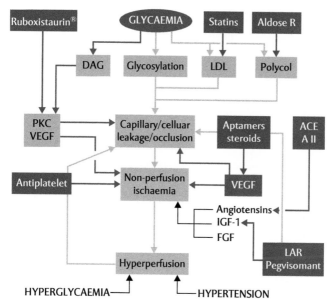

Aldose R = aldose reductase inhibitors
ACE = angiostensin converting enzyme
A II = angiostensin receptor II
DAG = diacyl glycerol
FGF = Fibroblast growth factor
IGF-1 = insulin-like growth factor 1
LAR = sandostatin LAR
(a somatostatin analogue)

LDL = low density lipoprotein
Pegvisomant = growth hormone
receptor antagonist
PKC = protein kinase C enzyme system
Ruboxistaurin® = selective inhibitor
of the β 1 & 2 isoforms of the protein
kinase enzyme system
VEGF = vascular endothelial
growth factor

Figure 16.4 Pathogenetic mechanisms in the development of DR. The two major mechanisms of vascular changes—hyperglycaemia and hypertension—and the biochemical pathways implicated in the pathogenesis of DR are illustrated.

Reproduced courtesy of Professor Paul M. Dodson and The Heart of England Retinal Screening Centre.

## 16.8 Summary

The medical management of patients with DR is focused on the proven benefit of tight glucose and BP control, with multiple cardiovascular risk factor intervention, including angiotensin receptor blockade, statin, and fibrate treatment. These aspects are still of paramount importance to patients in the early development of DR as well as for patients receiving ophthalmological treatments, including intravitreal therapies.

FURTHER READING

ACCORD Study Group and ACCORD Eye Study Group. (2010). Effects of medical therapies on retinopathy progression in type 2 diabetes. *New Engl J Med* **363**: 233–44.

Altaf QA, Dodson PM, Ali A, Raymond NT, Wharton H, Fellowes H, et al. (2017). Obstructive sleep apnoea and retinopathy in patients with type 2 diabetes. A longtitudinal study. *Am J Respir Crit Care Med* **196**(7): 892–900.

Brownlee M. (2001). Biochemistry and molecular cell biology of diabetic complications. *Nature* **414**; 813–20.

Chaturvedi N, Porta M, Klein R, Orchard T, Fuller J, Parving HH, et al. Effect of candersartan on prevention of retinopathy (DIRECT Prevent 1) and progression (DIRECT Protect 1) of retinopathy in type 1 diabetes: randomized, placebo controlled trials. *Lancet* **8**(373): 1394–402.

Chowdhury TA, Hopkins D, Dodson PM, Davies N. (2002). The role of serum lipids in exudative diabetic maculopathy: is there a place for lipid lowering therapy? *Eye* **16**: 689–93.

Colhoun HM, Betteridge DJ, Durrington PN, Hitman GA, Neil HA, Livingstone SJ, et al. (2004). Primary prevention of cardiovascular disease with atorvastatin in type 2 diabetes in the Collaborative Atorvastatin Diabetes Study (CARDS): multicentre randomized placebo-controlled trial. *Lancet* **364**: 685–96.

Diabetes Control and Complications Trial Group. (1993). The effect of intensive treatment of diabetes on the development and progression of long-term complications in insulin-dependent diabetes mellitus. *N Engl J Med* **329**: 977–86.

Donaldson M, Dodson PM. (2003). Medical treatment of diabetic retinopathy. *Eye* **17**: 550–62.

EUCLID Study Group. (1997). Randomised placebo-controlled trial of lisinopril in normotensive patients with insulin-dependent diabetes and normoalbuminuria or microalbuminuria. The EUCLID Study Group. *Lancet* **349**: 1787–92.

Ferris FL 3rd, Davis MD, Aiello LM. (1999). Treatment of diabetic retinopathy. *N Engl J Med* **341**: 667–8.

Gaede P, Vedel P, Larsen N, Jensen GV, Parving HH, Pedersen O, et al. (2003). Multifactorial intervention and cardiovascular disease in people with type 2 diabetes. *N Engl J Med* **348**: 383–93.

Gale R, Scanlon PH, Evans M, Ghanchi F, Yang Y, Silvestri G, et al. ( 2017). Action on diabetic macula oedema (DMO). *Eye* **31**: S1–20.

Joint British Society 2. (2005). Joint British Societies' Guidelines on prevention of cardiovascular disease in clinical practice. *Heart* **91**(suppl V): 1–52.

Keech AC, Mitchell P, Summanen PA, et al., for the FIELD study investigators. (2007). Effect of fenofibrate on the need for laser treatment for diabetic retinopathy (FIELD study): a randomised controlled trial. *Lancet* **370**(9600): 1687–97.

Nguyen QD, Tatlipinar S, Shah SM, Haller JA, Quinlan E, Sung J, et al (2006. ). Vascular endothelial growth factor is a critical stimulus for diabetic macular edema. *Am J Ophthalmol* **142**: 961–969.

Royal College of Ophthalmology. (2012). Diabetic retinopathy guidelines—DR Guidelines Expert Working Party. www.rcophth.ac.uk (accessed 21 August 2019).

Schmidt-Erfurth U, Garcia-Arumi J, Bandello F, Berg K, Chakravarthy U, Gerendas BS, et al. (2017). Guidelines for the management of diabetic macula oedema by the European Society of Retina Specialists (EURETINA). *Ophthalmologica* **237**: 185–222.

Sheetz MJ, King GL. (2002). Molecular understanding of hyperglycaemia's adverse effects for diabetic complications. *J Am Med Ass* **288**: 2579–88.

Sjolie AK, Klein R, Porta M, Orchard T, Fuller J, Parving HH, et al. (2008). Effect of candersartan on progression and regression of retinopathy in type 2 diabetes (DIRECT—Protect 2): a randomized placebo controlled trial. *Lancet* **372**: 1385–93.

UK Prospective Diabetes Study (UKPDS) Group. (1998). Intensive blood-glucose control with sulphonylureas or insulin compared with conventional treatment and risk of complications in patients with type 2 diabetes: UKPDS 33. UK Prospective Diabetes Study Group. *Lancet* **352**: 837–53.

UK Prospective Diabetes Study (UKPDS) Group. (1998). Tight blood pressure control and risk of macrovascular and microvascular complications in type 2 diabetes: UKPDS 38. UK Prospective Diabetes Study Group. *Br Med J* **317**: 703.

Wright AD, Dodson PM. (2011). Medical management of diabetic retinopathy: fenofibrate and ACCORD Eye studies. *Eye* **25**(7): 1–7.

# CHAPTER 17

# Patients of concern

Alexander D. Wright and Paul M. Dodson

---

**KEY POINTS**

- Worsening of retinopathy may be associated with:
- Rapid improvement in glycaemic control.
- Pregnancy.
- Hypertension.
- Renal failure.
- Being lost to follow-up.

---

## 17.1 Introduction

One of several factors may cause particular concern within a retinopathy screening programme, but the main categories are those patients whose glycaemic control improves rapidly, monitoring required during pregnancy, patients with hypertension, renal failure, and foot problems, and those patients who become lost to follow-up. Those lost to follow-up are considered in Chapter 13, 'Programme administration and fail-safe', but of special concern are patients attending renal and podiatry services, whose risk of retinopathy may go unnoticed.

## 17.2 Rapid changes in glycaemic control

Rapid improvement in glycaemic control may result in changes in refraction and in temporary worsening of retinopathy. Examples of situations where rapid changes in glycaemic control may occur are given in Box 17.1. In general terms, patients of concern due to improvement in glycaemic control should be screened prior to the change or new treatment, and 3 months later.

The reduction in HbA1c considered significant for worsening of retinopathy is not easy to define, as retinopathy is not always assessed when diabetes control is tightened. The Diabetes Complications and Control Trial in Type 1 diabetes showed a temporary worsening in the tightened control group (mean HbA1C reduced by 1.8%) with greater changes seen in those with poorest control.

A recent consensus meeting suggested that a reduction of HbA1C to be of concern was >2%, with some experts suggesting >3%.

> **Box 17.1** Examples of rapid changes in glycaemic control
>
> • Starting insulin (rarely other therapies).
> • Restarting insulin.
> • Starting an insulin pump in Type 1 diabetes.
> • Bariatric surgery for weight loss.
> • Islet cell/pancreas transplants.
> • New therapies for diabetes.

## 17.3 Clinical scenarios of concern

### 17.3.1 Bariatric surgery

Bariatric surgery (gastric banding or bypass) has been of particular concern because of the dramatic improvements in glucose tolerance achieved in some patients with diabetes and in some patients achieving a 'cure'. A recent report has assessed the impact of such surgery on the progression of diabetic retinopathy (DR) and the results were reassuring in that there was a lower progression to sight-threatening diabetic retinopathy (STDR) or maculopathy compared with those with non-surgical routine diabetic care. However, only a small number of patients achieved a reduction of >2%, so a major deterioration might not have been predicted. Nonetheless, screening prior to and 3 months after bariatric surgery seems prudent.

#### 17.3.1.1 Introduction of new therapies for diabetes

New therapies also have the potential to worsen diabetic complications, including DR. This was initially observed with worsening of retinopathy following the initiation of GLP 1 therapy in a patient with an initial HbA1C of 14% and subsequent reduction to 7%. It was difficult to be sure whether the retinopathy change was related to the drug therapy or the dramatic fall in HbA1C, the latter being the case after further patients were carefully screened prior to and after initiation of this therapy, with no evidence of deterioration.

#### 17.3.1.2 Initiation of insulin therapy or pump

Rapid changes in glycaemic control may be difficult to predict or influence, but should be considered, for example, in Type 2 diabetes when starting insulin, and in Type 1 diabetes when changing to a continuous infusion insulin pump. In all these circumstances, additional screening episodes should be considered.

## 17.4 Pregnancy

See Box 17.2.

> **Box 17.2** Guidance for retinal screening and pregnancy
>
> (Limited in UK to patients with pre-existing diabetes)
> - At pre-conception.
> - At booking-in all patients.
> - At 16–20 weeks gestation if not under eye clinic care.
> - At 28 weeks gestation in all patients.

Extra vigilance is advised during pregnancy, as retinopathy may deteriorate (NICE guideline NG3, updated August 2015) and data have confirmed the principles of this guidance. This vigilance should be extended to pre-conception care, when screening should be offered to women at their first appointment, unless they have had an annual retinal assessment in the previous 6 months. At the booking appointment in an established pregnancy, retinal screening should be offered to all patients with pre-existing diabetes, unless assessed in the previous 3 months. Pre-proliferative retinopathy and any form of referable retinopathy should be referred promptly and followed in the eye clinic. Further screening should be done at 16–20 weeks if background retinopathy *only* is found at the first antenatal visit, unless referral to ophthalmology had been arranged. Retinal screening should be offered in all pregnancies at 28 weeks' gestation, unless patients are already in ophthalmic care.

In view of these extra requirements, it is important to try and integrate pregnancy services closely with the retinal screening service to maximize uptake and ensure exchange of information. Retinal screening is not offered to patients with gestational diabetes in UK, as this group do not develop DR.

## 17.5 Renal failure

Renal failure is commonly due to diabetic kidney disease, where DR will be an accompanying feature that is likely to progress. Efforts should be made to ensure that patients and dialysis unit staff are aware of the need for continued eye screening by ophthalmology clinic services. The disruptive routine of renal dialysis 3 days a week may make clinic and screening appointments difficult to arrange care and, if not, to ensure appropriate screening. *In addition it should be noted that renal failure, anaemia, iron deficiency, blood transfusion, and erythropoietin treatment may all contribute to an unreliable measure of glycaemic control using HbA1C.*

### 17.5.1 Organ transplant

Newly diagnosed diabetes often occurs after organ transplantation, mainly due to the use of glucocorticoids and other anti-rejection drugs, all of which may precipitate diabetes, and are usually required on a permanent basis. Retinal screening should be arranged as soon as is practical as retinopathy may be present at the first screening. Screening should thereafter continue in the usual way.

With regard to pre-existing DR in patients undergoing pancreas or islet cell transplant, there is usually stabilization and reduction in progression over time, following a successful outcome

## FURTHER READING

Amin AM, Wharton H, Clarke M, Syed A, Dodson P, Tahrani AA. (2016). The impact of bariatric surgery on retinopathy in patients with Type 2 diabetes; a retrospective cohort study. *Surg Obes Relat Dis* **12**(3): 606–12.

Hamid A, Golar SK, Wharton H, Clarke M, Wright A. (2017). Diabetic retinopathy in newly diagnosed diabetes after kidney and liver transplantation. *Br J Diabet* **17**(1): 17–18. http://dx.doi.org/10.15277/bjd.2017.119 (accessed 21 August 2019).

Hampshire R, Wharton H, Leigh R, Wright A, Dodson P. (2018). Screening for diabetic retinopathy in pregnancy using photographic review clinics. *Diabet Med* **30**: 475–7.

Klefter ON, Hommel E, Munch IC, Nørgaard K, Madsbad S, Larsen M. (2016). Retinal characteristics during 1 year of insulin pump therapy in type 1 diabetes: a prospective, controlled, observational study. *Acta Ophthalmol* **94**(6): 540–7.

National Institute for Health and Care Excellence. (2016). Diabetes in pregnancy, Quality Standard QS 109. https://www.nice.org.uk/search?q=QS109 (accessed 21 August 2019).

Tekin Z, Garfinkel MR, Chon WJ, Schenck L, Golab K, Savari O, et al. (2016). Outcomes of pancreatic islet allotransplantation using the Edmonton protocol at the University of Chicago. *Transplant Direct* **2**(10): e105.

Thompson DM, Meloche M, Ao Z, Paty B, Keown P, Shapiro RJ, et al. (2011). Reduced progression of diabetic microvascular complication with islet cell transplantation compared with intensive medical therapy. *Transplantation* **91**(3): 373–8.

Zabeen B, Craig ME, Virk SA, Pryke A, Chan AKF, Cho YH, et al. (2016). Insulin pump therapy is associated with lower rates of retinopathy and peripheral nerve abnormality. *PLoS One* **11**(4): e0153033.

# Imaging in diabetic retinopathy

Sarita Jacob and Ramesh R. Sivaraj

---

**KEY POINTS**

- Imaging in diabetic retinopathy (DR) has developed over the years and the advantages are multifold.
- Optical coherence tomography (OCT) has revolutionized the management of diabetic maculopathy.
- Recent introduction of optical coherence tomography angiography (OCTA) has reduced the need for fundus fluorescein angiography (FFA) for macular ischaemia and proliferative retinopathy.
- Ultra-wide field (UWF) imaging modalities for colour fundus and FFA are very useful for documenting and assessing the overall retinal state and highlighting the periphery.

---

## 18.1 Colour fundus photographs

Digital fundus photography with mydriasis using two or three fields is commonly used by diabetic screening programmes. This is shown to have good specificity and sensitivity in comparison with the standard seven-field standard Early Treatment Diabetic Retinopathy Study (ETDRS) photography, which is too time-consuming with low patient compliance for screening. Patient compliance and comfort with screening is reasonably achieved with two-field fundus photography (see Chapter 10, 'The screening episode: visual acuity, mydriasis, and digital photography', and Chapter 11, 'How to grade').

## 18.2 Confocal scanning laser ophthalmoscopy and ultra-wide field imaging

Current screening methods with standard fundus photography lack the ability to image the periphery. Confocal scanning laser ophthalmoscopy (cSLO) and UWF imaging can be done without mydriasis, improving patient comfort and compliance further. cSLO uses a focused laser beam and captures the reflected light through a small aperture, producing a sharp high-contrast image. UWF imaging utilizes the principles of cSLO along with an ellipsoid mirror to capture wide-field images (100–200 degrees; see Figure 18.1) in comparison to standard fundus photograph (45 degrees). Commercially available systems presently using UWF technology

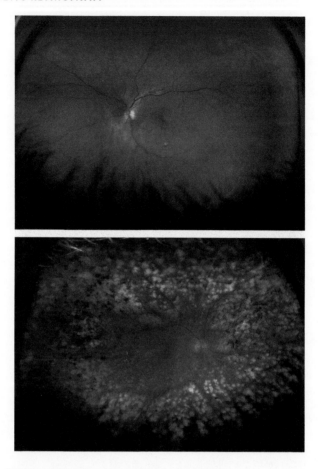

Figure 18.1 Examples of an ultra-wide field retinal image.

are the Optos retinal imaging and Heidelberg HRA. These systems can also be used for angiographic imaging with the use of appropriate filters. Limitations include eyelash artefacts and the inability to capture finer macular details.

Two-field views, as used in our screening protocol above, only visualize <20% of the total retina. Great potential can therefore be perceived of this photography in ophthalmology, but its place in screening is unclear at present, owing to the high cost compared with standard retinal cameras and the accuracy of macular assessment possible. Nevertheless, assessment of pre-proliferative DR and stable proliferative DR should be more accurate when compared with the standard screening two 45-degree photographs. Results of ongoing studies will no doubt clarify its role in the future.

CHAPTER 18

## 18.3 Fundus fluorescein angiography

This is a very useful and standard imaging modality for retinal vascular diseases, including diabetes, and has been used for many years. Sodium fluorescein is a water-soluble mineral-based dye which is injected intravenously. It is excited by blue light and emits or fluoresces yellow-green light. The dye leaks from damaged vessels when there is capillary endothelial damage, and from new vessels. It has been the gold standard to identify the source of leakage, areas of capillary non-perfusion (ischaemia) and neovascularization. In DR, FFA images show microaneurysms as punctate areas of hyperfluorescence and ischaemia is represented by patchy areas of hypofluorescence. An increase in the foveal avascular

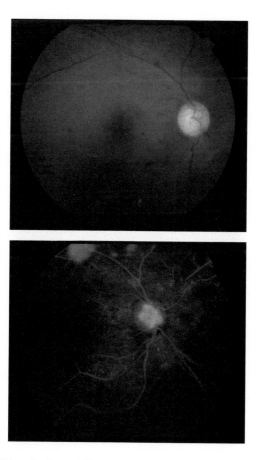

Figure 18.2 Colour fundus and FFA images showing NVD and NVE.

zone suggests macular ischaemia and accounts for visual loss in some patients (ischaemic maculopathy). Leakage of the dye occurs in the macula in diabetic macular oedema (DMO). It also identifies neovascularization on the optic disc (NVD) or new vessels elsewhere (NVE) characterized by leakage of the dye (Figure 18.2). Wide-field fluorescein angiography is now available with newer UWF systems, which help to identify capillary non-perfusion and ischaemia in the periphery and peripheral neovascularization. This is of great value in delivering targeted pan-retinal photocoagulation in proliferative DR. However, conventional FFA does have small risks owing to injection of the dye with allergic reactions and rarely anaphylaxis. This technique is less commonly used now with the advances in OCT and OCT-angiography (OCTA) described here.

## 18.4  Optical coherence tomography

OCT has, indeed, revolutionized the management of diabetic maculopathy, and is now the gold standard for diagnosis and monitoring of DMO. It is a non-invasive and non-contact technique which uses light to determine the optical reflectivity of retinal tissues. OCT systems have advanced considerably over the years since its inception. Initially, time domain (TD) technology was used, which was replaced by the faster spectral domain (SD) systems with better axial resolution and scanning speed. Newer technologies help in imaging the choroid as well either by enhanced depth imaging (EDI) or better depth penetration (Swept source). OCT in the current era can provide volumetric three-dimensional (3D) scans and complete retinal cross-sectional studies to assess all changes of diabetic maculopathy (see Figures 18.3–18.5). It is most useful in DR to confirm the diagnosis of oedema, exudates, cotton wool spots, drusen (see Figure 18.4), and macular traction.

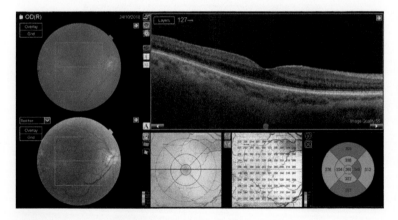

Figure 18.3  Normal OCT of the macula.

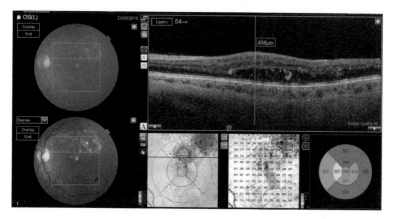

Figure 18.4 OCT showing exudates and oedema.

The intra-vitreal treatments with anti-VEGF or steroids for DMO are initiated and monitored with OCT measurements. OCT is also a logical investigation within the DR screening programme and particularly in the surveillance clinic pathway to identify those patients who have maculopathy according to screening criteria (M1) and macular oedema, and thus streamline referrals to eye clinics.

Recent studies have identified the value of the OCT in assessing the accuracy of the M1 criteria to predict macular oedema and cost effectiveness. They have

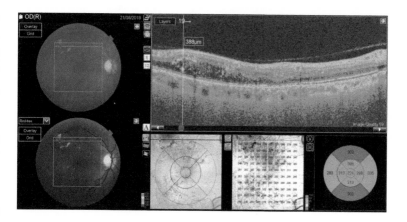

Figure 18.5 OCT showing exudates and oedema.

demonstrated that only 15–25% of patients with M1 have macular oedema, which allows 70% of M1 patients identified on screening to be followed-up by photography and OCT in a virtual clinic. This approach is now widely used within the UK screening programme. Studies are ongoing, investigating the cost effectiveness of such an approach, but initial studies have confirmed it is cost effective.

## 18.5 Optical coherence tomography angiography

This is a non-invasive motion contrast imaging modality, based on rapid OCT scanning of the eye comparing repeat scans acquired at the same position in the retina to interpret changes. In comparison with FFA, there are no risks associated with exogenous dye injection. There is rapid acquisition of images in seconds with in-depth resolution and assessment of the superficial and deep capillary plexus. OCTA can help to visualize microaneurysms, capillary non-perfusion, and neovascularization clearly without any dye injection (see Figures 18.6–18.8). This new imaging technique is, therefore, ideal for identifying neovascular activity in proliferative DR and macular ischaemia. Limitations include motion artefacts and a small field of view in comparison with conventional FFA.

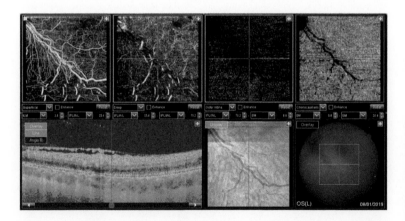

Figure 18.6 OCTA showing new vessels along the inferotemporal arcade (NVE).

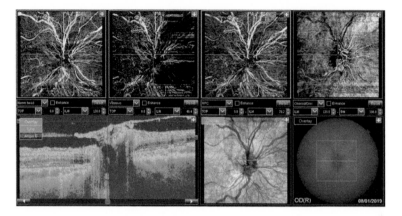

Figure 18.7 OCTA showing prolific new vessels on and above the optic disc (NVD).

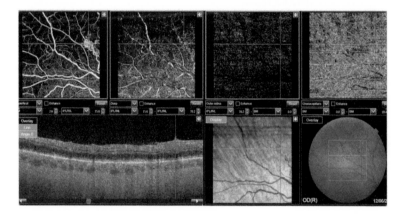

Figure 18.8 OCTA showing new vessels (NVE) superotemporally and Doppler flow showing red signal confirming activity of the new vessels.

## 18.6 B scan ultrasonography

This is a very useful imaging modality in proliferative DR in the presence of vitreous haemorrhage and media opacities, when the retina cannot be directly visualized by conventional methods of examination (see Figure 18.9). The B scan utilizes sound waves transmitted at a high frequency from a transducer and the amplitude

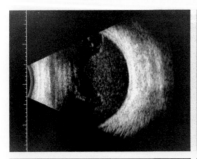
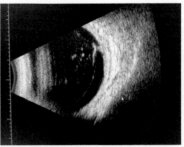

| B scan showing vitreous haemorrhage, which is predominantly subhyaloid and a flat retina | B scan showing early vitreo-retinal traction in a patient with vitreous haemorrhage |
| --- | --- |

Figure 18.9 Right, B scan showing early vitreo-retinal traction in a patient with vitreous haemorrhage. Left, B scan showing vitreous haemorrhage, which is predominantly subhyaloid, and a flat retina.

of signals reflected back from tissues is used to construct a two-dimensional (2D) image of the eye. This imaging is indicated to assess the retinal status to diagnose retinal tears, retinal detachment, and posterior vitreous detachment in the presence of vitreous haemorrhage, which prevents fundal view.

## 18.7 Artificial intelligence

Artificial intelligence (AI) based on deep learning (DL) is being studied in retinal imaging including 3D scans. Despite its limitations, this technology has the potential to revolutionize screening programmes and the practice of ophthalmology in the future.

FURTHER READING

De Fauw J, Ledsam JR, Romero Parades B, Nikolov S, Tomasev N, Blackwell S, et al. (2018). Clinically applicable deep learning for diagnosis and referral in retinal disease. *Nature Med* **24**: 1342–50.

Gajree S, Borooah S, Dhillon B. (2017). Imaging in diabetic retinopathy: a review of current and future techniques. *Curr Diabetes Rev* **13**(1): 26–34.

Goh JK, Cheung CY, Sim SS, Tan PC, Tan GS, Wong TY. (2016). Retinal imaging techniques for diabetic retinopathy screening. *J Diabetes Sci Technol* **10**(2): 282–94.

Kashani AH, Chen CL, Gahm JK, Zheng F, Richter GM, Rosenfeld PJ, et al. (2017). Optical coherence tomography angiography: a comprehensive review of current methods and clinical applications. *Prog Retin Eye Res* **60**: 66–100.

Leal J, Luengo-Fernandez R, Stratton IM, Dale A, Ivanova K, Scanlon PH. (2018). Cost-effectiveness of digital surveillance clinics with optical coherence tomography versus hospital eye service follow-up for patients with screen-positive maculopathy. *Eye (Lond)* **33**(4): 640–7.

Prescott G, Sharp P, Goatman K, Scotland G, Fleming A, Philip S, et al. (2014). Improving the cost-effectiveness of photographic screening for diabetic macular oedema: a prospective, multi-centre, UK study. *Br J Ophthalmol* **98**(8): 1042–9.

Salz DA, Witkin AJ. (2015). Imaging in diabetic retinopathy. *Mid E Afr J Ophthalmol* **22**(2): 145–50.

Scanlon P. (2018). Digital surveillance with OCT and the treatment of diabetic macular oedema. *Diabet Eye J* **11**: 6–11.

Staurenghi G, Sadda S, Chakravarthy U, Spaide RF. (2014). International Nomenclature for Optical Coherence Tomography (IN•OCT) panel. Proposed lexicon for anatomic landmarks in normal posterior segment spectral-domain optical coherence tomography: the IN•OCT consensus. *Ophthalmology* **121**(8): 1572–8.

Ting DSW, Pasquale LR, Peng L, Campbell JP, Lee AY, Raman R, et al. (2019). Artificial intelligence and deep learning in ophthalmology. *Br J Ophthalmol* **103**(2): 167–75.

# CHAPTER 19

# Ophthalmic treatment of diabetic retinopathy

Ramesh R. Sivaraj and Jonathan M. Gibson

---

**KEY POINTS**

- Laser photocoagulation remains a cost-effective option for the treatment of diabetic retinopathy (DR), either alone or in combination with pharmacotherapy.
- Recent advances in laser technology allow quicker, more accurate, and safer treatment.
- Vitreo-retinal surgery has an important role in cases of advanced DR.
- Cataract surgery in diabetic patients with retinopathy requires careful pre-operative assessment and may require special treatment regimes.

---

The optimal treatment strategy for DR requires management of the underlying diabetes mellitus and associated risk factors, and ophthalmic management is aimed at preserving vision. Ideally, this is best achieved when patients are managed with close co-operation between the diabetic and ophthalmic teams, with good access to the images from the DR screening programme.

The ophthalmologist has an important educational role to give feedback of findings and progress of patients to the referring screening programme, and to referring general practitioners (GPs), diabetic physicians, and optometrists. In this manner, the whole service benefits by a two-way flow of information.

The management of DR is a fast-moving field and, for an excellent overview, the reader is recommended to visit the Royal College of Ophthalmologists guidelines, which are updated at regular intervals.

The treatments available are discussed under the following headings:

- *Retinal laser treatment*: used for proliferative diabetic retinopathy (PDR) and diabetic macular oedema (DMO) in different strategies.

- *Pharmacotherapy*: administration of drugs by intra-vitreal or peri-ocular routes. (This important subject will be discussed in Chapter 20, 'New treatment strategies for diabetic eye disease'.)
- Treatment for advanced diabetic retinal disease by pars plana vitrectomy.
- Treatment of patients with cataracts and DR.

## 19.1 Retinal laser treatment

For many years retinal laser photocoagulation was the only proven treatment that was available for the treatment of DR. However, despite new developments in intra-vitreal pharmacotherapy for DR, laser photocoagulation remains an important treatment modality for DR. It is available in all ophthalmic units, is quick to perform by a skilled operator, and is highly cost-effective.

LASER is an acronym for 'light amplification by stimulated emission of radiation'. Unlike white light, laser light is composed of one wavelength and is coherent, meaning that the light waves are all in phase. Both these properties make lasers highly focusable and, for treatments of the retina, the light energy is absorbed by the retinal pigment epithelium, producing a thermal reaction (photocoagulation).

The vast majority of treatments are performed on an outpatient basis, using a slit lamp with a laser attachment. A special contact lens is applied to the patient's cornea after local anaesthesia drops are instilled, and this allows a stereoscopic view to be obtained of the fundus. Different lenses are available for treatment of maculopathy with pan-retinal photocoagulation (PRP), depending on the angle of view and magnification required. An additional benefit of the lenses is that they very effectively help to control inadvertent movement of the patient's eye.

## 19.2 Treatment for proliferative retinopathy

Laser PRP for DR has been shown to be an effective treatment for sight preservation in PDR (see Figure 19.1). This has been confirmed in a number of important clinical trials.

The Diabetic Retinopathy Study (DRS) was an important landmark trial that provided the main evidence-base for laser treatment in PDR (DRS Research Group, Report no. 8, 1981). The DRS was a prospective multicentre clinical trial, which showed that scatter laser photocoagulation reduced the risk of severe visual loss by at least 50%. It also confirmed that argon laser and xenon light coagulation were equally effective, but that harmful effects were more common with xenon, and this led to the widespread introduction of argon laser facilities into eye departments.

Scatter laser or PRP is indicated for PDR when retinal new vessels elsewhere (NVE) or new vessels at the optic disc (NVD) are present, and are considered at risk of bleeding (see Figures 19.2 and 19.3). The aim of PRP is to destroy the areas where there is capillary non-perfusion and retinal ischaemia, thereby reducing the

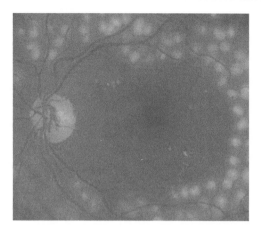

Figure 19.1 Fresh scatter laser PRP reactions after laser photocoagulation with 532-nm frequency doubled YAG laser. Note the NVD.
Reproduced courtesy of Professor Paul M. Dodson and The Heart of England Retinal Screening Centre.

formation of growth factors, which are powerful stimulants to new vessel production. In most eyes, this will mean an application of over 2000 retinal burns of spot-size 500 μm, or more if the burns are smaller. It is customary in most units to fractionate this treatment into two sessions, which is more comfortable for the patient and is less associated with side effects. In this way, treatment sessions are

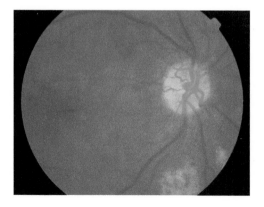

Figure 19.2 Patient with NVD and NVE. Previous laser scars are visible.
Reproduced courtesy of Professor Paul M. Dodson and The Heart of England Retinal Screening Centre.

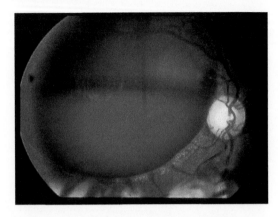

Figure 19.3 **Large pre-retinal haemorrhage in patient with PDR.**
Reproduced courtesy of Professor Paul M. Dodson and The Heart of England Retinal Screening Centre.

able to be completed in about 10–15 minutes, although with newer technologies, such as the patterned-scanning laser (PASCAL), this is considerably quicker.

## 19.3 Diabetic maculopathy

The great advances in retinal imaging have enabled many patients with mild to moderate DMO that is not considered sight-threatening to be serially monitored by means of optical coherence tomography (OCT) and fundus imaging, and does not require treatment unless it becomes necessary. However, when treatment is required, the main choice is between focal laser photocoagulation or injection of intra-vitreal or peri-ocular drugs, or increasingly a combination of treatments.

Laser treatment has been used as the first line of treatment for DMO for over 40 years. The Early Treatment Diabetic Retinopathy Study (ETDRS) was a large prospective multicentre clinical trial, which showed that prompt laser treatment of clinically significant macular oedema (CSMO) can reduce the risk of visual loss by one half (ETDRS Research Group, Report no. 1, 1985). It also showed that, while visual improvement was unlikely, laser treatment was effective in preventing further visual loss.

The introduction of intra-vitreal pharmacotherapy has been found to be highly effective in the treatment of DMO and, being non-destructive to the retina, has largely replaced laser treatment as a stand-alone treatment for DMO. However, laser and intra-vitreal pharmacotherapy may be combined in specific cases of diabetic maculopathy.

The advent of OCT has revolutionized the assessment and treatment of DMO, and allows for precise targeting of treatment and monitoring of effect. It is considered in more detail in Chapter 18, 'Imaging in diabetic retinopathy'.

## 19.4  Side effects of laser treatment

Laser retinal treatment is destructive, however, and like all treatments has potential side effects.

- Laser PRP can be uncomfortable for the patient. This is dependent on the duration and power of the laser burns, the amount given, the position in the fundus, and the wavelength of the laser energy. Most new lasers allow much shorter exposures to be given than conventional DRS and ETDRS parameters, while still being effective, and generally, nowadays, there is no reason for laser PRP to be uncomfortable for the patient.

- Vitreous haemorrhage may occur after laser PRP if there are extensive fronds of NVE present, and this is thought to be due to contraction and bleeding from the fronds.

- Worsening of macular oedema following laser PRP is well recognized and is thought to occur as a decompensation of the macular capillaries, probably due to alteration in macular blood flow following PRP. It can be prevented by fractionating laser PRP to smaller numbers of burns and by performing laser treatment for maculopathy before PRP. Increasingly, anti-vascular endothelial growth factor (anti-VEGF) injections are being administered before or after laser PRP.

- Inadvertent foveal burn may occur if there is sudden uncontrolled patient movement during laser treatment or if the operator becomes disorientated with fundus landmarks. It is usually a catastrophic event for both patient and operator, giving rise to immediate and permanent loss of central vision. Fortunately, it is extremely rare and most ophthalmic units would never encounter a case, but it is wise to be constantly aware of its possibility.

- Loss of peripheral vision and reduction in night vision may occur if extensive PRP is given. This may have important implications for the patient if they are a motor vehicle driver, particularly if it is required as part of their employment. It may be a necessary risk for the patient to accept this as a means of maintaining vision, but it should be discussed with the patient prior to PRP being carried out. With newer laser technology and less collateral damage, this is less common than in previous years when very heavy peripheral laser treatment was given.

## 19.5 Advances in laser technology

With advances in technology the earlier gas lasers have now been replaced by solid state laser machines, which are based on diode laser technology. This means that they are considerably more robust and energy efficient than the earlier models, and are extremely compact and portable. This latter point is important for cases that may be treated in outpatients, as well as in the operating theatre.

The latest advances have been the introduction of micropulse laser technology in which the retinal laser reactions are kept to a minimum to avoid collateral damage to the healthy functioning retina, thereby lessening visual loss from laser treatment. Advances have also been made in the use of pattern application of laser burns, by which multiple laser reactions in the retina, set to a predetermined pattern, are achieved by a single application. This is the basis of semi-automated retinal PASCAL, which enables much quicker PRP treatments to be developed than conventional treatment. The NAVILAS laser system (navigated laser) is another new development, whereby digital images are used to plan and deliver precise laser treatments.

## 19.6 Surgery for advanced diabetic retinopathy

Pars plana vitrectomy is a specialized procedure, which is the domain of highly trained, specialist, ophthalmic surgeons. Vitrectomy surgery is used to achieve specific goals, which may limit or halt the progress of advanced diabetic eye disease.

These are:

- To remove vitreous opacity (commonly vitreous haemorrhage, also intra-ocular fibrin, or cells) and/or fibrovascular proliferation (severe extensive proliferative retinopathy, anterior hyaloidal fibrovascular proliferation).
- To allow completion of PRP laser (with the endo-laser introduced into the vitreous cavity, or with the indirect laser ophthalmoscope) or direct ciliary body laser photocoagulation in cases of neovascular glaucoma.
- To relieve retinal traction, and traction retinal detachment by removal or dissection of epi-retinal membranes.
- To achieve retinal reattachment by closure of breaks and placement of internal tamponade (in cases of retinal detachments).
- To remove the posterior hyaloid face in some cases of diffuse macular oedema with posterior hyaloid face thickening.

Vitrectomy surgery now allows many cases of advanced DR to be salvaged with resultant retention of vision. Surgery can be performed under local anaesthesia as a day case, but for prolonged procedures, general anaesthesia may be preferable.

## 19.7 Treatment of cataracts in the diabetic patient

Cortical and posterior subcapsular cataracts are associated with diabetes, and cataract prevalence increases with the duration of diabetes and is linked with poor diabetic control. Patients with diabetes are more likely to develop cataracts at an earlier age and cataracts are likely to progress faster than in the non-diabetic population.

Surgery is commonly indicated if the patient's vision is beneath the level required for driving or if fundus visualization is poor. Modern cataract surgery in the diabetic patient is highly successful, although it is associated with an increased risk of ocular complications.

Small incision phacoemulsification with a foldable lens implant is the preferred current option and surgery is performed as a day case with local anaesthesia. Generally, if laser treatment is required it is best to perform this prior to cataract surgery if possible, but if visualization of the fundus is difficult due to the cataracts, laser treatment can be applied per-operatively, with the indirect ophthalmoscope, or post-operatively, within a few days.

DR may progress more rapidly after cataract surgery and it is, therefore, advisable to monitor the eyes closely for progression of DR, and in cases with severe retinopathy, early review is advisable.

FURTHER READING

DRS Research Group. (1981). Photocoagulation treatment of proliferative diabetic retinopathy: clinical applications of Diabetic Retinopathy Study findings. DRS report number 8. *Ophthalmology* **88**: 583–600.

ETDRS Research Group. (1985). Photocoagulation for diabetic macular edema: Early Treatment Diabetic Retinopathy Study, Report Number 1. *Arch Ophthalmol* **103**: 1796–806.

Royal College of Ophthalmologists Diabetic Retinopathy Guidelines. (2012, updated 2013). Eye to eye podcast. www.rcophth.ac.uk (accessed 21 August 2019).

CHAPTER 20

# New treatment strategies for diabetic eye disease

Sobha Joseph and Ramesh R. Sivaraj

**KEY POINTS**

- Argon laser treatment was the mainstay of treatment for diabetic retinopathy (DR) and maculopathy up to the last decade.
- Anti-vascular endothelial growth factors (anti-VEGFs) and steroid implants have revolutionized treatment outcomes.
- Newer long-acting drugs are likely to be available soon.

## 20.1 Introduction

Advances in research in the last decade have led to the development of newer treatments for DR. There is now a better understanding of the underlying pathology of diabetic macular oedema (DMO). It has been shown that increased permeability of damaged capillaries, leading to macular oedema, occurs not only from hypoxia, but also from inflammatory processes expressing inflammatory markers like cytokines in the retinal tissues. Moreover, neurodegenerative changes also contribute to the process of increased retinal vascular permeability.

The VEGFs induced by hypoxia cause increased capillary permeability and macular oedema. In proliferative DR and DMO, vitreous VEGF levels are noticeably high. Anti-VEGF drugs, which block the receptors for VEGF, have been developed and have become the mainstay of treatment for central foveal-involving macular oedema. Furthermore, in most cases of chronic macular oedema, anti-inflammatory, slow-release steroid implants are effective in improving and preserving vision. These treatments are given as intra-vitreal injections by an ophthalmologist or by trained practitioners, in a clean room as a sterile procedure.

## 20.2 Anti-vascular endothelial growth factors for diabetic macular oedema

There are two anti-VEGF drugs approved in the UK for DMO involving the centre of the macula. They have been approved for treatment of macular oedema of 400 μm or more (see Figure 20.1):

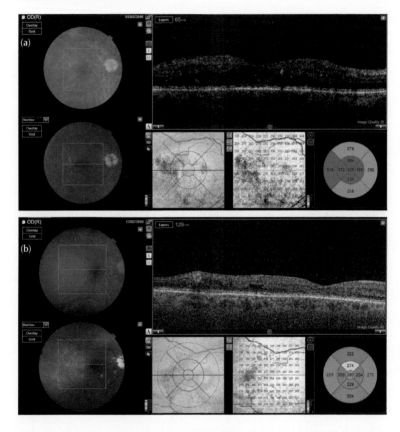

Figure 20.1 (a,b) Macular scans demonstrating improvement in macular oedema following a course of anti-VEGF treatment (note irregular and thin retina indicating damage to the retina despite resolution of oedema).

- *Ranibizumbab (Lucentis) 0.5 mg*: a monoclonal VEGF A inhibitor, given as monthly intra-vitreal injections until visual acuity is stabilized. Treatment is resumed if vision deteriorates during monthly monitoring. It has been shown that most patients may need up to seven injections in the first year. Treatment can be extended up to 3 months if the treat-and-extend pathway is followed.
- *Aflibercept (Eylea) 2 mg*: a VEGF receptor fusion protein, which combines with VEGF A, B, and placental growth factor. It is given as five monthly injections and then every 2 months in the first year. The treatment interval

can be extended in the second year based on the vision and clinical response.

- *Bevacizumab (Avastin)*: has shown similar efficacy in DMO and, while in use in countries primarily owing to lower cost, it is not licensed in the UK for DMO treatment.

Contraindications to the anti-VEGF agents are mainly ocular or peri-ocular infections, and hypersensitivity to the drugs. Although rare, infection (0.05–0.1% of injections performed), retinal tear, vitreous haemorrhage, lens injury, inflammation, and increased intra-ocular pressure are the most significant side effects. Patients may develop a subconjunctival haemorrhage following injection or experience floaters from posterior vitreous detachment.

## 20.3 Steroids for diabetic macular oedema

Slow-release steroid implants inhibit the inflammatory markers in the retina and also have some anti-VEGF properties. Dexamethasone and fluocinolone acetonide are the two licensed steroid implants in the UK, which can be used in pseudophakic eyes with chronic macular oedema (see Figure 20.2). The main side effects are increased eye pressure and cataract formation. Therefore, treated patients need regular intra-ocular pressure monitoring. The drug has been approved for use only in pseudophakic eyes.

- *Dexamethasone (700 μg)*: intra-vitreal implant (Ozurdex) slowly releases the steroid over a period of 4–6 months before dissolving completely. It is licensed for use in chronic DMO, when other treatments are unsuitable or ineffective. It can be repeated after 6 months if the patient notices worsening of vision due to recurrence of macular oedema.
- *Fluocinolone acetonide (190 μg)*: intra-vitreal implant (Iluvien) is a sustained-release, non-biodegradable micro-implant, which releases 0.2 μg/day for approximately 36 months. It has anti-inflammatory and anti-VEGF properties.
- *Peri-ocular or intra-vitreal triamcinolone acetonide*: has been used for DMO in the past.

The actions of anti-VEGF and steroid implants are not long-lasting. Thus, some patients may require additional *macular laser* treatment as an adjuvant treatment. Macular non-perfusion is not a contraindication for these intra-vitreal treatments, although there is a subset of patients who are non-responsive to any of the currently available intra-vitreal treatments, despite changing intra-vitreal anti-VEGF agents or steroids.

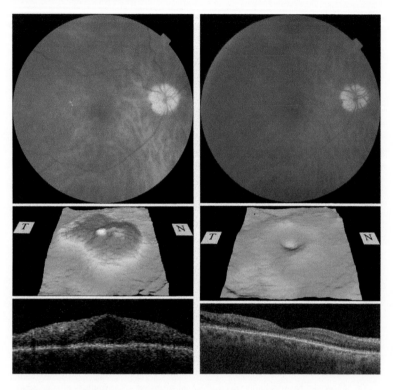

Figure 20.2 (a,b) DMO pre- and post-fluocinolone acetonide injection. (The topography map uses warm colours such as red and orange to indicate elevation/oedema.)

## 20.4 Proliferative diabetic retinopathy

Pan-retinal photocoagulation (PRP) is still the standard treatment for proliferative diabetic retinopathy (PDR) (see Chapter 19, 'Ophthalmic treatment of diabetic retinopathy'). However, recent studies have shown that monthly ranibizumab is comparable in efficacy to laser treatment in the management of PDR and it is especially beneficial if the proliferative retinopathy is associated with DMO. The Diabetic Retinopathy Clinical Research Network (DRCR net) has performed studies and demonstrated that, in patients with PDR, visual acuity outcomes were similar in those who are ranibizumab- or PRP-treated, after 5 years of study. Vision-threatening DMO and visual field loss was less in the ranibizumab treatment group, although patient-reported outcomes were similar in both groups, a factor to consider when choosing the treatment. These data support the efficacy of anti-VEGF injections in PDR, but they are not currently licensed for use in PDR in the UK. Other factors to consider in the choice of treatment include potential compliance with multiple hospital visits, cost, and general health.

Other non-licensed uses of anti-VEGF are in the treatment of anterior segment neovascularization (termed iris neovascularization or iris rubeosis, see Chapter 4, 'Diabetes and the eye,' Figure 4.5) and prior to vitrectomy for vitreous haemorrhage in PDR.

## 20.5 Drugs in development

- *Abiciparpegol* (anti-VEGF DARPin inhibitor) has a longer half-life in the vitreous and may reduce the frequent need for treatment.
- *AKP-9778* given subcutaneously and combined with ranibizumab has shown a reduction in DMO by increasing the phosphorylation of Tie2 (tyrosine kinase receptors) in the angiopoietin/Tie2 pathway in clinical trials.
- *RO6867461* is a biphasic immunoglobulin with one arm binding to VEGF and the other to Ang-2.
- *Inhibitors of plasma* kallikrein, integrin, and vascular adhesion protein- 1 (VAP-1) are under clinical trials.

## 20.6 Summary of management of diabetic macular oedema and proliferative diabetic retinopathy

- *Central involving DMO*: anti-VEGF (ranibizumab or aflibercept) monthly or bi-monthly treatment with or without macular laser.
- *Chronic DMO*: steroid implants if other treatments not suitable or not effective.
- *Non-centre involving clinically significant macular oedema*: macular laser.
- *PDR*: PRP.
- *PDR with significant DMO*: anti-VEGF and PRP.
- *PDR with iris neovascularization*: anti-VEGF and PRP.
- *Non-clearing vitreous haemorrhage*: vitrectomy with or without anti-VEGF.
- *Tractional retinal detachment/epi-retinal membrane (ERM)*: vitreo-retinal surgery.

FURTHER READING

BMJ Best Practice. The re-invention of best practice. https://bestpractice.bmj.com (accessed 22 August 2019).

Diabetic Retinopathy Clinical Research Network. (2010). Randomized trial evaluating ranibizumab plus prompt or deferred laser or triamcinolone plus prompt laser for diabetic macular edema. *Ophthalmology* **117**: 1064–77.

Gross JG, Glassman AR, Liu D, Sun JK, Antoszyk AN, Baker CW, et al. (2018). Diabetic Retinopathy Clinical Research Network. Five-year outcomes of pan retinal photocoagulation vs intravitreous ranibizumab for proliferative diabetic retinopathy: a randomized clinical trial. *J Am Med Ass Ophthalmol* **136**(10): 1138–48.

Miller K, Fortun JA. (2018). Diabetic macular edema: current understanding, pharmacologic treatment options, and developing therapies. *Asia Pacif J Ophthalmol (Phil)* **7**(1): 28–35.

National Institute for Health and Care Excellence. Improving health and social care through evidence-based guidance. https://www.nice.org.uk (accessed 22 August 2019).

Royal College of Ophthalmologists. Clinical guidelines. https://www.rcophth.ac.uk/standards-publications-research/clinical-guidelines/ (accessed 22 August 2019).

# Appendix

## A1.1 Screening intervals

At the time of writing, many countries have embarked on a national diabetic eye screening programme (DESP) using digital imaging. These include the Netherlands, Finland, Sweden, Norway, Portugal, Spain, Southern Ireland, and Denmark. Other countries have advanced systems in place, including France, Germany, Italy, and the Czech Republic. Outside Europe, New Zealand and Singapore have established national screening for diabetic retinopathy (DR), and there are advancing systems in the UAE, and Australia. Other countries use other modalities of screening, including ophthalmologists, e.g. in the USA. There are also a number of programmes based in Africa now reporting data on success.

It is not surprising that there are differences in systems and pathways according to individual countries' care systems. There does seem to be agreement on the principle of extended the screening intervals in Europe, with most schemes adopting 2- or even 3-yearly screening for those who exhibit no symptoms of DR. While there are abundant data to support this approach, there are practical issues in implementation with changes required to software and patient education.

## A1.2 Diabetic retinopathy grading systems

The primary aim of the national screening programme for DR in the UK is to detect diabetic eye disease at a stage at which vision loss can be limited by laser and other treatments. A working party for England and Wales was convened, and reported the minimum data set of retinopathy grades as four levels (R and M grades) in 2003, as described in previous chapters. However, the most common grading system used around the world is that suggested by the American Academy of Ophthalmology for the USA, which is based on the Early Treatment of Diabetic Retinopathy Study (ETDRS) using seven-field stereoscopic retinal photography. This grading system is used in research studies and has levels of 10 through to 85, termed mild non-proliferative (levels 10–35), moderate to severe non-proliferative (levels 43–53), high-risk proliferative to advanced proliferative DR (levels 61–85; see Table A1).

This system has been considered too complicated for routine clinical use in screening in the UK, and it does not define referable maculopathy in retinal images well. The UK has, therefore, continued with the classification of background, pre-proliferative, and proliferative retinopathy, and maculopathy, given R and M grades, respectively. A number of countries are using a hybrid of the UK and USA systems, reporting on the level of retinopathy by the EDTRS system, and maculopathy by the UK M grading system.

The two grading systems are compatible as shown in Table A2.

Of importance to the treatment of maculopathy, the ETDRS study observed benefit in those that it defined as having 'clinically significant macular oedema' (CSMO). The definitions are complicated, but the essence is the presence of exudates and retinal

**Table A1** DR disease severity scale and international clinical DR disease severity scale

| Disease severity level | Findings observable upon dilated ophthalmoscopy |
| --- | --- |
| No apparent retinopathy | No abnormalities |
| Mild NPDR | Microaneurysms only |
| Moderate NPDR | More than just microaneurysms, but less than severe NPDR |
| Severe NPDR | |
| USA definition | Any of the following (4-2-1 rule) and no signs of proliferative retinopathy:<br>• Severe intra-retinal haemorrhages and microaneurysms in each of four quadrants<br>• Definite venous beading in two or more quadrants<br>• Moderate IRMA in one or more quadrant |
| International definition | Any of the following and no signs of proliferative retinopathy:<br>• More than 20 intra-retinal haemorrhages in each of four quadrants<br>• Definite venous beading in two or more quadrants<br>• Prominent IRMA in one or more quadrants |
| PDR | One or both of the following:<br>• Neovascularization<br>• Vitreous/pre-retinal haemorrhage |

IRMA, intra-retinal microvascular abnormalities; NPDR, non-proliferative diabetic retinopathy; PDR, proliferative diabetic retinopathy.

*Note:* Any patient with two or more of the characteristics of severe NPDR is considered to have very severe NPDR. PDR may be classified as high-risk and non-high-risk.

Source: Reproduced from American Academy of Ophthalmology Retina/Vitreous Panel. Preferred Practice Pattern®Guidelines. Diabetic Retinopathy. San Francisco, CA: American Academy of Ophthalmology; 2017. Available at: www.aao.org/ppp. Copyright © 2014 American Academy of Ophthalmology. Source data from Wilkinson CP, Ferris FL III, Klein RE, et al. Proposed international clinical diabetic retinopathy and diabetic macular edema disease severity scales. *Ophthalmology* 2003;110:1679.

thickening at or within 500 μm of the macula centre (i.e. fovea), or one disc area of retinal thickening within one disc diameter (1DD) of the macula centre. Current European guidelines emphasize the importance of differentiating macular oedema into central and non-central foveal involvement for treatment paradigms, rather than using CSMO.

## A1.3 Visual acuity scales

The visual acuity scale described in Chapter 10, 'The screening episode: visual acuity, mydriasis, and digital photography', uses the Snellen and LogMAR charts. There

## Table A2 EDTRS grading

| EDTRS grading (based on seven-field photography) | | |
|---|---|---|
| 10 | DR absent | R0 |
| 20 | MAs only | |
| 35 | Mild, non-proliferative | |
| 43 | Moderate NPDR | R2 |
| 47 | Moderately severe NPDR | |
| 53 | Severe NPDR | |
| 61, 65, 71, 81 | Proliferative DR | R3 |
| DR, diabetic retinopathy; MA, microaneurysm; NPDR, non-proliferative DR. | | |

are differences across the globe in visual scales used with the Snellen (feet), Snellen (metre), decimal, and LogMAR recordings. In particular, the research studies use either LogMAR or the decimal method, and Snellen (feet) is used in clinical practice in the USA. Table A3 shows the values and comparative values of the different systems.

## Table A3 The approximate values of visual acuity on the different scales used across Europe and the USA

| Snellen (feet) | Snellen (m) | Decimal | LogMAR |
|---|---|---|---|
| 20/200 | 6/60 | 0.10 | 1.00 |
| 20/160 | 6/48 | 0.13 | 0.90 |
| 20/120 | 6/36 | 0.17 | 0.78 |
| 20/100 | 6/30 | 0.20 | 0.70 |
| 20/80 | 6/24 | 0.25 | 0.60 |
| 20/60 | 6/18 | 0.33 | 0.48 |
| 20/50 | 6/15 | 0.40 | 0.40 |
| 20/40 | 6/12 | 0.50 | 0.30 |
| 20/30 | 6/9 | 0.63 | 0.18 |
| 20/25 | 6/7.5 | 0.80 | 0.10 |
| 20/20 | 6/6 | 1.00 | 0.00 |
| 20/16 | 6/4.8 | 1.25 | −0.10 |
| 20/12 | 6/3.6 | 1.67 | −0.22 |
| 20/10 | 6/3 | 2.00 | −0.30 |

# Index

Tables, figures, and boxes are indicated by an italic t, f, and b following the page number.

*For the benefit of digital users, indexed terms that span two pages (e.g., 52–53) may, on occasion, appear on only one of those pages.*